MEDIATORS OF INFLAMMATION

CONTRIBUTORS

Ira M. Goldstein Department of Medicine, Division of Rheumatology, New York University School of Medicine, New York, New York

Peter M. Henson Department of Experimental Pathology, Scripps Clinic and Research Foundation, La Jolla, California

David A. Levy Johns Hopkins Medical Institutions, Baltimore, Maryland

Shaun Ruddy Department of Medicine, Medical College of Virginia, Virginia Commonwealth University, Richmond, Virginia

Jocelyn Spragg Department of Medicine, Harvard Medical School, and Department of Medicine, Robert B. Brigham Hospital, Boston, Massachusetts

Daniel J. Stechschulte Department of Medicine, University of Kansas Medical Center, Kansas City, Kansas

Gerald Weissmann Department of Medicine, Division of Rheumatology, New York University School of Medicine, New York, New York

Robert B. Zurier Department of Medicine, University of Connecticut School of Medicine, Farmington, Connecticut

MEDIATORS OF INFLAMMATION

Edited by

Gerald Weissmann

Department of Medicine
Division of Rheumatology
School of Medicine
New York University Medical Center.
New York, New York

PLENUM PRESS · NEW YORK AND LONDON

Library of Congress Cataloging in Publication Data

Weissmann, Gerald.
  Mediators of inflammation.

  Includes bibliographies and index.
  1. Inflammation. I. Title. [DNLM: 1. Inflammation. QZ150 W433m]
RB131.W44   616'.047   74-20786

ISBN-13: 978-1-4684-0747-1   e-ISBN-13: 978-1-4684-0745-7
DOI: 10.1007/978-1-4684-0745-7

© 1974 Plenum Press, New York
Softcover reprint of the hardcover 1st edition 1974

A Division of Plenum Publishing Corporation
227 West 17th Street, New York, N.Y. 10011

United Kingdom edition published by Plenum Press, London
A Division of Plenum Publishing Company, Ltd.
4a Lower John Street, London W1R 3PD, England

PREFACE

Lewis Thomas has suggested that "Perhaps the inflammatory reaction should be regarded as a defense of an individual against all the rest of nature, symbolizing his individuality and announcing his existence as an entity." Provision of these symbols and announcements is the task of various mediators of inflammation and this volume has been designed to present our current understanding of their biochemistry, cellular origins, pharmacology, and role in pathology. Unlike other volumes of collected papers, this book did not result from a specific conference or symposium at which each contributor presented his own, narrowly framed research experience. Rather, each of the chapters represents, in the form of a general review, a summary of our knowledge of the mediators and the mechanisms by which they are released to launch the inflammatory response. Much effort has been taken to insure that the often conflicting terminology in this field is defined in detail: many synonyms (e.g., of the properdin system or the alternate pathway of complement activation) have been repeatedly presented, in order to avoid confusion. Although each of the contributors is actively engaged in the field of inflammation, few text figures or tables of ongoing research have been included; the overall aim was to provide a volume readily accessible to workers in other areas as well as to the general reader.

It can now be appreciated that the study of inflammation and its mediators has passed from the purely descriptive to the soundly quantitative level of analysis, and it is hoped that this compact volume will conveniently bring the results of this effort to the attention of biologists, biochemists, immunologists, pathologists, and clinicians. Scrutiny of the chapters will indicate that they represent views of inflammation currently held in New York, Boston, Hartford, Kansas City, Baltimore, Richmond, and La Jolla; the editor would especially like to thank Drs. Charles G. Cochrane and K. Frank Austen for suggestions as to their contents.

This volume was prepared during tenure by the editor of a Guggenheim

Fellowship at the Centre de Physiologie et d'Immunologie Cellulaires at the Hospital St. Antoine in Paris and thanks also are due to Dr. Roger Robineaux for his hospitality. Ms. Sarah Cohen prepared the index, Dr. Sylvia Hoffstein provided the cover figure, and Mrs. Harriet Funt contributed her invaluable secretarial help.

New York   G. W.

CONTENTS

Chapter 1

MECHANISMS OF MEDIATOR RELEASE FROM INFLAMMATORY CELLS
Peter M. Henson

Chapter 2

LYSOSOMAL HYDROLASES AND INFLAMMATORY MATERIALS

Ira M. Goldstein

Chapter 3

THE PLASMA KININ-FORMING SYSTEM
Jocelyn Spragg

Chapter 4

THE COMPLEMENT AND PROPERDIN SYSTEMS

Shaun Ruddy

Chapter 5

HISTAMINE AND SEROTONIN

David A. Levy

Chapter 6
PROSTAGLANDINS
Robert B. Zurier

Chapter 7
SLOW REACTING SUBSTANCES
Daniel J. Stechschulte

MEDIATORS OF INFLAMMATION

INTRODUCTION

Gerald Weissmann

There is probably no such thing as a general "inflammatory process" during which a variety of carefully programmed cells release, or act on, a carefully sequenced series of inflammatory mediators. Probably there are as many varieties of inflammation as there are inflammatory stimuli. Consequently, this volume will be directed toward an analysis of the *mediators* of inflammation, with the implicit assumption that one or another of these is more "important" in one or another sort of inflammation. As Lewis Thomas (1971) has pointed out, the inflammatory response may well have been devised as a means of keeping even the lowliest of organisms safe from outside invaders or fusion to its fellows in a kind of pan-syncytium. Thus when we try to understand how complex organisms handle physical injury, foreign organisms, or immune injury, we are confronted with an exercise in biological archeology. Moreover, our analysis seems destined to have become couched in military terms: "defense" and "attack," "invasion" and "retreat," "injury" and "loss."

At each step of the evolutionary ladder, organisms have added to or modified existing ways of waging this microscopic warfare. Consequently, when we begin to describe the outlines of any specific inflammatory event we are likely to encounter remnants of very primitive responses among the very latest defensive techniques. Thus chemotaxis is recognized in bacteria, unicellular organisms phagocytose and release lysosomal enzymes, complement developed before teleosts, and cyclic nucleotides and prostaglandins modulate cell functions in

GERALD WEISSMANN Department of Medicine, Division of Rheumatology, New York University, New York, New York.

animals without backbones. But mammals use each of these means (and more) to cope with foreign material or injury.

Therefore, it is not easy to give a "general" outline of an inflammatory cycle, and to discuss a common sequence of cells and mediators which form its circumference. What can be done, however, is to look at chemically identified mediators of inflammation and to study how these appear in various discrete types of inflammation. It is this approach that has been used in this volume.

1. THE MEDIATORS OF INFLAMMATION

There are several ways of classifying these mediators of inflammation: thus histamine, serotonin, SRS-A, kinins, and prostaglandins have been called "imme-

Table I. Mediators of Inflammation

Agent	Chemical nature	Origin
1. Histamine; serotonin	Amine (stored)	Basophil, mast cell; platelets
2. Slow reacting substance of anaphylaxis (SRS-A)	Acid lipid	Leukocyte
3. Kinins	Polypeptides (split products)	Plasma substrate
4. Prostaglandins	Acid lipids (newly synthesized)	Ubiquitous intra-cellular precursors
5. Plasmin	Protease (split product)	Plasma substrate (liver)
6. Hageman factor (activated)	Protease	
7. Complement	Plasma proteins and split products	Reticuloendothelial cells, liver
8. Lysosomal enzymes	Intracellular proteins (stored)	PMNs, macrophages, mast cells
9. Lymphokines	Intracellular proteins (newly synthesized)	Stimulated lymphocytes

diators" by virtue of their appearance early in inflammation and in the lesions of immediate hypersensitivity. Complement and lysosomal enzymes have been called "intermediators" because they appear somewhat later, but this is the most arbitrary of divisions. In Table I, I have listed the most important mediators of inflammation, and, of course, the most noticeable aspect of this list is that it points out omissions from this volume. Thus, for example, it is clear that elements of the blood-clotting system (especially Hageman factor) and the fibrinolytic system (plasmin) have crucial roles in launching or amplifying early inflammation. However, the chapters on kinins and complement clearly indicate the possible role of these proteins of clotting and lysis in the sequences of limited proteolysis that accompany activation of the kinin and complement cascades. But perhaps the greatest omission is that of the various lymphocyte factors, or "lymphokines," which clearly mediate the later stages of immune tissue injury. Inclusion of these would probably have doubled the length of this volume. Nor has there been included a separate chapter on chemotaxis. I would classify this biological activity, not as the property of any distinct group of mediators, but as one shared by several others of the well-characterized mediators such as complement (e.g., C5a, C3a), lysosomal enzymes (neutral protease, cathepsin D), and perhaps even the prostaglandins (of the E and F series).

2. MECHANISMS COMMON TO SEVERAL MEDIATOR SYSTEMS

It is, however, possible to discern among the various trails leading to acute inflammation at least five general pathways which seem to be shared by more than one system of mediation. These are as follows:

2.1. Cellular Release

By mechanisms which bear more than a coincidental resemblance to other secretory processes, cells respond to injury, phagocytosable particles, or immune challenge by releasing previously stored or inactive substances. Examples are the release of histamine and SRS-A from lung tissue, histamine from mast cells or blood basophils, and lysosomal enzymes from polymorphonuclear leukocytes.

2.2. Fluid-Phase Activation

Surface injury to cells or supporting structures (e.g., basement membrane), as well as exposure to immune complexes, leads to activation in the fluid phase (plasma or tissue) of coordinated, limited proteases which generate mediators by cleaving precursor substrates readily available in these fluids. Examples are the cleavage of C3 by the activation of early complement components or the properdin system, the activation of prekallikrein to kallikrein by activated Hageman factor, and the cleavage of kininogens by kallikrein to form kinins.

2.3. Bypass Mechanisms

Factors, usually proteases, released from cells or activated in the fluid phase can bypass earlier steps in the activation sequence of fluid-phase mediators. Examples are the cleavage by lysosomal enzymes of C3 or C5, the direct activation of kinins by leukocyte kininogenases, and the generation of separate C3 and C5 cleaving enzymes by the properdin system.

2.4. Extracellular Control Loops

Some mediators of inflammation inhibit or amplify steps leading to their own elaboration. Examples are the inhibition of histamine release by histamine, the enhanced release of lysosomal enzymes (some of which can cleave C5 to C5a) by C5a, the activation by plasmin of Hageman factor which may itself be used to generate more plasmin, and the requirement for C3b in the properdin-mediated activation of C3PAase (factor D).

2.5. Intracellular Controls

Perhaps the greatest degree of similarity is discerned among substances released from cells. It has recently been appreciated that cAMP or substances which lead to its intracellular accumulation (β-adrenergic agents, histamine, prostaglandin E_1) *inhibit* release of histamine from leukocytes or lung fragments, lysosomal enzymes from polymorphonuclear leukocytes or macrophages, and lymphokines from stimulated lymphocytes. In contrast, cGMP or substances which lead to its intracellular accumulation (cholinergic agents, prostaglandin $F_{2\alpha}$) *enhance* release of histamine from leukocytes or lung fragments, lysosomal enzymes from polymorphonuclear leukocytes, and lymphokines (Fig. 1). Moreover, good circumstantial evidence implies that the cyclic nucleotides exert their effects by virtue of their as yet undefined interaction with microtubules. Thus assembly of tubules (as in D_2O) is associated with *enhanced* release or histamine or lysosomal enzymes, and disassembly (as by colchicine or vinblastine) *diminishes* release of histamine or lysosomal enzymes. It is in this framework that one can understand the intracellular effects of the anaphylatoxin C5a, which en-

YIN / YANG HYPOTHESIS OF MEDIATOR RELEASE

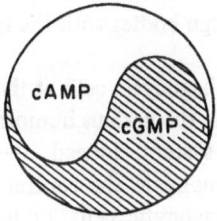

SECRETION ↓ BY cAMP	SECRETION ↑ BY cGMP
Lysosomal enzymes	Lysosomal enzymes
Histamine	Histamine
SRS-A	SRA-A
Lymphokines	Lymphokines

Fig. 1. Yin/yang hypothesis of mediator release.

hances lysosomal enzyme release, assembles microtubules, and provokes chemotaxis. In contrast, histamine and prostaglandins of the E series inhibit their own further elaboration by raising cAMP levels within leukocytes. Finally, it is clear that Ca^{2+} ion is required for most forms of mediator release.

3. CENTRALITY OF PHAGOCYTES

But before committing ourselves to detailed analysis of feedback loops, amplification systems, and interactions between cells and the fluid phase, let us recall some of the simplification that Metchnikoff (1905) introduced into this area in the 1800s. He correctly formulated that there is no phagocytosis without inflammation and almost as correctly proclaimed the validity of the reverse of that statement. In considering that phagocytosis is at the critical center of the inflammatory response, he was influenced by his own fight with the humoral school of Cohnheim and Ehrlich. Since Celsus, it had been clear that *rubor, calor, tumor,* and *dolor* led to *laesio functio.* But the humoral school taught that the various circulating substances which mediated redness, heat, swelling, and pain were brought to the injured site by capillaries, the function of which was at the center of inflammation. Metchnikoff, by training a zoologist, was able to show that inflammation (accumulation of phagocytes, swelling of the area, and tissue injury) took place in cold poikilotherms, so that fever was not necessary, and proceeded to demonstrate that anesthetized limbs underwent inflammation, showing that pain was unnecessary. But even more convincing was the finding that tissues without capillaries (the sclerae) or animals without a vascular system (starfish larvae) reacted to foreign bodies with the influx of phagocytes, swelling, and tissue injury.

These observations place phagocytic cells at the center of inflammation, and suggest, to me at any rate, that the various humoral mediators are in themselves only a sort of amplification system. Indeed, the acquisition of vascular and immune systems seems to complicate the central interaction of inflammation: the release, by injured or phagocytic cells, of inflammatory materials. If we begin with this interaction as the critical point, we can go on to appreciate that tissue injury and *laesio functio* must result from the attack, by substances released from phagocytic cells, of substrates which are critical for the function of cells and connective tissue. Now for extracellular structures to be injured, we require hydrolysis of covalent bonds by enzymes; for cell membranes the problem is complicated by the fact that the lipid bilayers of biomembranes can undergo dissolution in the presence of amphipathic molecules in the absence of enzymatic attack (Sessa *et al.*, 1969).

Consequently, it seems reasonable to suggest that only those mediators which can actually cleave covalent bonds in connective tissue (lysosomal hydrolases) or which can act as amphipaths (terminal components of the complement sequence) can be held responsible for irreversible tissue injury. In contrast, the other mediators would appear to be responsible for the earlier and potentially reversible aspects of inflammation. Thus kinins, prostaglandins, histamine, and the early components of complement equip injured or invaded tissue with the responses of vasodilatation, capillary leakage, chemotaxis, and the accumulation of leukocytes. Indeed, it is the general finding that animals or humans genetically deficient in Hageman factor (i.e., chickens or Mr. Hageman) or in complement components still manage to mount adequate inflammatory responses. In contrast, absence of polymorphonuclear cells seems to diminish tissue responses to injury to a much greater degree. Therefore, and the prejudices of the editor are obvious, the response of inflammation can be viewed as resulting from the release by injured and/or phagocytic cells of substances which eventually serve a protective role, although initially provoking a nasty effect. These substances, reacting with circulating materials, activate several cascades of limited proteolysis in tissue fluids which amplify the limited capacity of individual cells. Since some of the products of inflammation (e.g., histamine or prostaglandin E_1) in turn inhibit further release of mediators, the response may be viewed as biphasic or cyclic.

If the following series of chapters serve their intended function, they should provide occasional experimental evidence in favor of the outline provided above, but, more likely, they will probably convince the reader that any such general theory or description of "inflammation" is probably as premature as a general theory of behavior.

4. REFERENCES

Metchnikoff, E., 1905, *Immunity in Infective Diseases,* reprinted by Johnson Reprint Corp., New York and London (1968).

Sessa, G., Freer, J. H., Colacicco, G., and Weissmann, G., 1969, *J. Biol. Chem.* 244:3575.

Thomas, L., 1971, in: *Immunopathology of Inflammation* (B. K. Forscher and J. C. Houck, eds.), p. 1, Excerpta Medica, Amsterdam.

MECHANISMS OF MEDIATOR RELEASE FROM INFLAMMATORY CELLS

1

Peter M. Henson

1. INTRODUCTION

The inflammatory process is manifested by cell and tissue changes which are in large measure produced by mediating substances derived from various cells or plasma sources. The mediators have the general character that in the normal state they exist as precursors or are sequestered in sites where they are inactive. Stimuli which initiate the inflammatory response then activate or induce synthesis of the mediators or lead to their release. It is this release of mediators from cells which is the subject of this chapter.

A variety of cells in the body contain potent mediators of inflammation and in addition, in some instances, inhibitors for the control of the inflammatory process. Those cells which have been most studied for their mechanisms of

This is publication No. 779 from the Department of Experimental Pathology, Scripps Clinic and Research Foundation, 476 Prospect Street, La Jolla, California 92037.

This work was supported in part by the U.S. Public Health Service Grant GM 19322-02. Dr. Henson is the recipient of a U.S. Public Health Service Career Development Award (5 K04 GM 42567-04).

PETER M. HENSON Department of Experimental Pathology, Scripps Clinic and Research Foundation, La Jolla, California.

release of mediators include mast cells, basophils, platelets, neutrophils (poly-morphonuclear neutrophil leukocytes, PMNs), and to a lesser extent macro-phages and lymphocytes. The release processes clearly fall into two categories: (a) *cytotoxic release,* where for a variety of reasons the cell is destroyed and its content of mediators is thereby liberated, and (b) *noncytotoxic release,* where the mediators are actively secreted. There are remarkable similarities between the secretory processes in the different cells, and this release of mediators bears a striking resemblance to secretory phenomena in general (see Becker and Henson, 1973; Stormorken, 1969). An additional emphasis in this chapter will be on the possibilities of interaction between different cells to initiate the liberation of more mediators.

The mediators are characteristically confined within intracytoplasmic gran-ules, and the cells fall into three types characterized by the type of granule and mode of secretion. *Mast cells, basophils,* and *platelets* have morphologically similar dense granules containing potent vasoactive amines (histamine and/or serotonin) probably bound ionically, and these appear to be released by similar mechanisms. *Neutrophils* and *macrophages* have lysosomes which contain many potential mediators including proteolytic enzymes. Finally, *lymphocytes* appear to generate a number of mediators, the lymphokines (David and David, 1972). While the origin and mechanism of release of the lymphokines are largely unknown, evidence is accumulating that lymphocyte stimulation may induce synthesis of mediators, followed by a process resembling the secretory reactions described below (Henney and Bubbers, 1973; Plaut *et al.,* 1973). Lymphocytes (particularly when activated) also contain lysosomes (see Weissmann and Dukor, 1970) but not in large quantity, and it is not clear whether these may be released to the outside of the cell and, if they are, what significance this may have. In addition, mediators in other cells (e.g., endogenous pyrogen in neutrophils, Bodel, 1970) may be synthesized *de novo* following appropriate stimulation of the cell.

At the outset, a general problem in the study of mediator release can be mentioned—the homogeneity of the cell populations being investigated. This problem arises in all aspects of such studies, namely, the location of the mediator in a particular cell type, the interaction of the stimulus with the mediator-containing cell, the release process, and the effect of inhibitors on the reactions. This will be particularly evident in the discussion of the controlling influence of cAMP on release (see below). In some cases, purified cells can be obtained (platelets, neutrophils). In others, while purified cells are available (rat peritoneal mast cells, mouse peritoneal macrophages) there is a risk that these represent unique populations of the cells, so that generalizations from them may be invalid.

Most of the experimental data on release of mediators have been obtained *in vitro* with isolated cells or tissue fragments. Nevertheless, some information is available which ties the *in vitro* observations to *in vivo* inflammatory reactions. In many disease situations, the triggering pathogenetic event is unknown. Yet understanding the processes of mediation of tissue injury can nevertheless allow prevention of the damage if inhibitors of the mediators or of their release are known. Consequently, emphasis on natural or artificial inhibition is important.

The field of release of mediators is growing with extreme rapidity, and while it is now possible to probe the cellular mechanisms involved, nevertheless many problems remain to be solved before the processes described can be defined in molecular terms. Some current theories will be presented, which should help to define the processes as they are known and to indicate some of the thinking of investigators working in this area. Since the literature on mediator release is vast, the references section is in no way complete. Reviews will often be cited, in particular the recent and more detailed discussion of *in vitro* release of mediators by Becker and Henson (1973).

2. GENERAL CHARACTERISTICS OF MEDIATOR RELEASE FROM CELLS

By definition, noncytotoxic release (secretion) involves liberation of granule contents but not of constituents from the cytoplasm (cf. Section 2.6). The release will first be discussed in general terms and then some properties of the individual cell types will be considered.

2.1. Mediators

Mediators vary widely from cell to cell and are primarily contained within membrane-bound, intracytoplasmic granules.

2.2 Morphology of the Noncytotoxic Release Process

The granules must in some way discharge their contents to the outside of the cell. Although not completely understood, in some cells (e.g., neutrophils) this appears to involve migration of granules to the plasma membrane, fusion of granule membrane with plasma membrane, and discharge of contents (i.e., a process of exocytosis). In other cells (e.g., mast cells), movement of granules is less evident and propagated fusion of granule membranes occurs (with some eventual extrusion of granules). In still others (e.g., basophils), it is not clear how the granules gain access to the exterior.

2.3. Stimuli for Noncytotoxic Release

Stimuli for noncytotoxic release vary widely between the different mediator-containing cells. They all appear to act at the external surface membranes, which suggests the presence on the cells of receptors (often specific) for the different stimuli (see Section 2.4.1). Some general groups of stimuli may be mentioned: (a) Immunoglobulins are a stimulus for all the cells discussed. Although the class of immunoglobulins may vary for each cell type, they all interact with specific cell-surface receptors by the Fc portion of the molecules. (b) For many of the cells, a variety of low molecular weight positively charged peptides or proteins (e.g., complement-derived anaphylatoxins) are stimuli. (c) A number of the cells respond to certain proteolytic enzymes (e.g., platelets to thrombin, mast cells to chymotrypsin). (d) In addition, a further source of stimuli for release is cell–cell interaction (e.g., between basophils and platelets). Many of these stimuli have been identified *in vivo* as well as *in vitro*.

The presentation of stimulus on a surface, or as a particle, in many cases increases its effectiveness (e.g., for neutrophils, macrophages, or platelets). In any case, there is increasing evidence for the requirement that the stimulus be at least divalent, although whether this is true of the low molecular weight activators as well is as yet unknown. This may indicate a requirement for aggregation of receptors in the cell membrane.

2.4. Mechanisms of Noncytotoxic Release

The exact mechanisms involved in the steps between stimulus and secretion (stimulus–secretion coupling, see Douglas, 1968) are still unknown. Nevertheless, some of the participating factors and controlling influences are recognized. A discussion of these should serve (a) to outline the cytological processes involved, (b) to compare them with those in other cells and with other cell functions in the same cell, and (c) to suggest possible therapeutic approaches to abrogation of the release of inflammatory mediators.

2.4.1. Serine Esterases. Increasing evidence suggests the involvement of cell-bound esterases (proteases) in the release of mediators. Release from most of the cells is inhibited in the presence of diisopropyl fluorophosphate (DFP) and a variety of phosphonate inhibitors (Becker and Henson, 1973). Pretreatment of either the stimulus or the cells with the inhibitors (which irreversibly inhibit serine esterases) followed by washing generally does not prevent a subsequent release from the cells reacting with the stimulus. Such data have been used to postulate the presence of an activatable (precursor) serine esterase on or in the cells, which is activated by the stimulus and only then becomes susceptible to the irreversible DFP inhibition. Such an enzyme has been demonstrated directly in neutrophils (Becker, 1972).

Activation of precursor serine esterases is a possible way in which cell reactions, including release, may be initiated (triggered). Use of the phosphonate inhibitors, which exhibit specific activity—structure profiles in inhibiting different known serine esterases such as thrombin, trypsin, and chymotrypsin, suggests that in many cases different stimuli activate different esterases on one cell type. This may reflect different cell-surface receptors. If the process indeed represents a cell-activating mechanism, the ability of added esterases (e.g., trypsin) to induce release from the cells might be explained in one of two ways: Such esterases might act on the substrate in the cell normally cleaved by the cell enzymes which are activated by the various stimuli. Alternatively, the esterases might activate the proenzymes, as trypsin is known to activate many proesterases (Fig. 1).

A similarity between the proposed serine esterase mechanism for activation of these cells and the known processes by which the complement and coagulation systems are initiated is suggested. A precursor serine esterase (C1 or Hageman factor) is activated (presumably by conformational changes) by interaction with a di- or multivalent stimulus. The activated esterase then initiates (by limited proteolysis) a series of molecular events leading to complement fixation or coagulation, respectively. This situation may be analogous to stimuli interacting at the cell surface. Many such stimuli appear to be di- or multivalent.

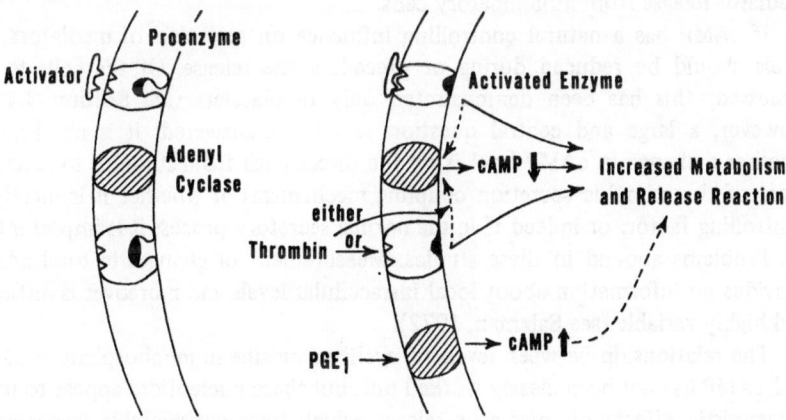

Fig. 1. Proposed stimulation mechanism for noncytotoxic release from mediator cells involving activation of a proesterase which triggers the secretory process. The enzyme might also temporarily inhibit adenylate cyclase (broken arrows) to reduce cAMP and remove the inhibitory (controlling) influence of the nucleotide.

Crosslinking receptors (receptor aggregation) or crosslinking sites on one receptor molecule may induce the necessary changes (perhaps conformational) to expose an enzymatic site. This can then initiate a chain of events leading to the various cell activities, including release of mediators (Fig. 1).

2.4.2. Divalent Cations. Ca^{2+} in the external medium is generally required for release, as it is for many secretory phenomena (Rubin, 1970). A few exceptions may be related to mobilization of internal sources of Ca^{2+} since prolonged preincubation with EGTA can, even in these situations, prevent the release. The relative concentrations of Ca^{2+} and Mg^{2+} may also be important. Recently, penetration of Ca^{2+} into mast cells has in fact been shown to trigger the secretory reaction (Foreman *et al.*, 1973) and in muscle cells to induce contraction (Levy *et al.*, 1973). This emphasizes the similarities between secretion and muscle contraction (see Becker and Henson, 1973).

2.4.3. Cyclic Nucleotides. Cyclic 3',5'-adenosine monophosphate (cAMP) appears to play an important role in the release of mediators, but precisely what role is not yet clear. Generally, addition of the nucleotide, or of agents which increase its intracellular levels, inhibits release. Conversely, mechanisms for specifically decreasing the levels enhance release. Phosphodiesterase inhibition (e.g., by methylxanthines) or adenylate cyclase stimulation (e.g., by PGE_1) induces the former. β-Adrenergic agents generally stimulate adenylate cyclase, and this increases intracellular cAMP and also inhibits secretion. α-Adrenergic stimulation, on the other hand, decreases the activity of adenyl cyclase in some cells, and this may enhance the release reaction. In general, cAMP is inhibitory in mediator release from inflammatory cells.

If cAMP has a natural controlling influence on secretion of mediators, its levels should be reduced during or preceding the release. Of the cells to be discussed, this has been demonstrated only in platelets (see Section 3.4.3). However, a large and central question remains unanswered: it is not known whether a change in cAMP level is on the direct path from stimulus to reaction (part of the stimulus–secretion coupling mechanism) or whether it is merely a controlling factor, or indeed if in the normal secretory process it is important at all. Problems abound in these studies. Measurement of changes in total cAMP provides no information about local intracellular levels and moreover is difficult and highly variable (see Salzman, 1972).

The relationship between levels of cyclic guanosine monophosphate (cGMP) and cAMP has not been clearly worked out, but these nucleotides appear to have antagonistic effects on mediator release which have considerable importance (Kaliner *et al.*, 1972; Goldberg *et al.*, 1973; Zurier *et al.*, 1974). Thus cholinergic agents may increase cGMP, and this appears to enhance the release process, opposing the action of cAMP. The interrelationship of Ca^{2+} and cAMP (Rasmussen, 1970) and that of Ca^{2+}, cAMP, and microtubules (Gillespie, 1971) are also highly significant. Although cAMP-dependent protein kinases have been de scribed in platelets and neutrophils, their nature and function have not yet been ascertained. Nevertheless, despite these important provisos it is possible to suggest that cAMP and perhaps cGMP exercise a controlling influence on the release (see Section 3.4.3. and Fig. 1). Evidence does seem to indicate that in these particular cells cAMP does not act as the simple "second messenger" originally advocated by the enormously important work of Sutherland and his associates (see Robison et al., 1971).

2.4.4. Energy Metabolism. Secretion is an energy-requiring process, and the ATP is supplied by different pathways in different cells.

2.4.5. Microtubules. Microtubules appear to play a role in secretion as seen morphologically and through the inhibitory action of the specific microtubule-disrupting agent colchicine (see Olmstead and Borisy, 1973; Taylor et al., 1973). How they contribute is not clear. There is suggestive evidence that they act in directing motion either of the whole cell or of granules within the cell (e.g., Freed and Lebowitz, 1970). Thus it is possible that they serve to direct the granule toward the stimulated external membrane with which it then interacts. It is also becoming evident that microtubules may act as a "cytoskeleton" and serve to maintain or contribute to cell shape (e.g., of platelets). Contractile elements may in fact act on the microtubules as muscles do on bones or may act in opposition (McGuire and Moellmann, 1972). A colchicine-binding protein (perhaps microtubular) has also been linked with the mechanism of surface receptor aggregation and perhaps with cell-membrane stimulation (Ukena and Berlin, 1972). Ca^{2+} and cAMP may also be involved in microtubule function (Gillespie, 1971). Moreover, cyclic GMP, in enhancing mediator release, appears to exert this effect by influencing assembly of microtubules (Goldstein et al., 1973; Zurier et al., 1974).

2.4.6. Contractile Protein. Actinomyosinoid material is present in most cells, including those containing mediators. In some cells, this has been distinguished morphologically as microfilaments. It has been suggested that such contractile elements are intimately involved in secretion and that their action may in part comprise the Ca^{2+} and ATP requirements (see Section 2.4.2). Perhaps the microfilaments move granules around in the cytoplasm. More probably they may normally prevent access of granules to membrane and by contracting allow this to occur more readily. There is some highly speculative evidence for this, in that cytochalasin B, thought to act by disrupting microfilaments (Wessels et al., 1971), seems to allow greater movement of granules and enhances secretion from neutrophils. However, cytochalasins may have a number of other actions and their use as a specific probe for microfilaments is coming under question. Changes in cell volume have also been demonstrated to follow stimulation, although since these must also involve ion and water fluxes, whose possible role is not at all understood, it is uncertain as yet what significance the observations have.

2.4.7. ATPases and Sulfhydryl Groups. Mediator release from many of the cells appears to involve ATPases. In some cases these may be Na^{2+} dependent, as evidenced by ouabain inhibition. Presumably, if contractile proteins are involved, Ca^{2+}-dependent ATPases may also play an important role in release. Sulfhydryl reagents, which inhibit ATPases, prevent release from all the cells studied but may act on so many proteins that their use does not serve at the moment to clarify the release process (Becker and Henson, 1973).

2.4.8. Synthetic Processes in the Cells. In most cases discussed here, synthesis of mediators is not involved; they are prepackaged. Neither does protein synthesis seem to be required. However, increased turnover of phospholipid is associated with cell stimulation.

2.4.9. Membrane Fusion. A little understood but integral part of the secretory phenomenon is the fusion between granules and external membranes. Many suggestions as to mechanism have been made, including the possible involvement of lysolecithin, Ca^{2+}, triphosphoninositide, and positively charged proteins (see Becker and Henson, 1973; Lucy, 1971; Woodin and Wieneke, 1970).

2.4.10. Order of Interaction. By reversibly inhibiting the secretory process and testing other inhibitors or inhibitory conditions for their effect before and after the reversibly inhibited step, it is possible to begin to piece together a sequence of events involved in release. Generally it has been found that the putative esterase activation is a very early step and precedes the steps modulated by cAMP. Energy requirement is generally late in the reaction sequence.

2.4.11. Inhibitors and Control of Release. Some potential inhibitors have been indicated in the preceding sections. Thus a large group of inhibitors act by increasing intracellular levels of cAMP. Another group may act on the cell membrane. Some drugs (e.g., aspirin) may act by altering prostaglandin synthesis (Vane, 1971). *In vivo,* release of prostaglandins may act as an important controlling influence on mediator liberation as well as to supply possible mediators (the prostaglandins themselves). Corticosteroids are also important inhibitors of the reactions.

PGE_1 and methylxanthines (e.g., caffeine and theophylline) inhibit release from most of the cells discussed, and in some cases this has been shown *in vivo* as well as *in vitro.* Other inhibitors (e.g., aspirin and disodium chromoglycate) appear to act more specifically on particular cells (e.g., platelets and mast cells, respectively. The potential for such specific inhibition of one cell or even one cell function emphasizes the importance of understanding the release mechanisms. An interesting phenomenon which may act as a feedback control is the recently demonstrated inhibition of basophil release by histamine, the material released (Lichtenstein and Gillespie, 1973).

Neurohormonal control of release of inflammatory mediations may be extremely important. Thus cholinergic drugs enhance the release in a number of systems, probably as a result of increasing cGMP in the cells. In contrast, adrenergic agents tend to alter cAMP levels and control release in this way.

Another source of inhibitors and controls affects the stimulus to the cells. Most of the potent stimuli which have *in vivo* significance are effectively controlled in the animal, so that their action does not proceed unchecked. These would include the inhibition of C3a by serum carboxypeptidase, of C3b by C3b-inactivator, of the platelet-activating factor from basophils by unknown serum proteins, and of the action of aggregated immunoglobulin (or complexes) on platelets and neutrophils by free immunoglobulin in excess.

Finally, inhibitors may be present, or administered, which prevent the action of the mediators themselves. For example, α_1-antitrypsin and colloidal gold inhibit neutrophil proteases.

2.5. Cytotoxic Reactions

Cytotoxic reactions are evidenced by liberation of cytoplasmic enzymes, peptides, and amino acids and disruption of the cell membrane. While many materials can induce lysis of cells *in vitro*, it is probable that *in vivo* the mechanisms are more limited. In the presence of complement, antibody directed against the cell is highly cytotoxic. Other complement-dependent reactions may involve some of the cells (e.g., platelets) as "innocent bystanders." Neutrophils phagocytose materials (e.g., urate crystals) which can cause lysis from within.

2.6. Release In Vivo

The cells discussed have almost all been shown to release mediators *in vivo* under some circumstances. This has provided support for the extensive *in vitro* study of the mechanisms involved. Evidence has included morphological observation (mast cells), detection of particular mediators (neutrophils), or specific depletion of the cells in question (platelets, neutrophils). Evidence for the involvement *in vivo* of a number of the stimuli described is accumulating for each cell type, for example, by specific depletion of complement. Cytotoxic reactions also occur *in vivo*, both specifically mediated (e.g., by complement) and nonspecifically mediated, when factors leading to necrosis cause liberation of mediators from any of the mediator cells which may be involved.

3. PLATELETS

Mammalian blood platelets exhibit a variety of activities which are potentially of great importance to inflammatory reactions. Predominant among these is the "release reaction" (Grette, 1962), i.e., the noncytotoxic release of platelet granule constituents. However, the related activities of adhesion, aggregation, and generation of coagulation cofactors may also participate in tissue injury. Platelet reactions may be considered in three phases. Platelets first adhere to particles or surfaces, or bind a soluble stimulus. Following the *adherence* (adhesion) is the *release* reaction, in which constituents are liberated. Among them is ADP, which itself causes *aggregation* (platelets binding to platelets) of more platelets, which may themselves now release mediators. If the initial stimulus was multivalent, it may also crosslink platelets, but this agglutination is distinguishable from true aggregation, in which the mechanism is still unknown.

Throughout the platelet cytoplasm are spaces, the canalicular system, which connect with the external milieu (White, 1971). The platelet may thus be likened to a sponge, and a large number of plasma proteins have been shown to be closely associated with it. This property may play an important role in inflammatory reactions, providing a highly favorable environment for activation of plasma enzyme systems such as the coagulation, complement, kinin-forming, and fibrinolytic systems. It would be accentuated by the recruitment of new platelets as a result of the reaction of complement or thrombin, which themselves can cause platelet adhesiveness, aggregation, and release (Fig. 2).

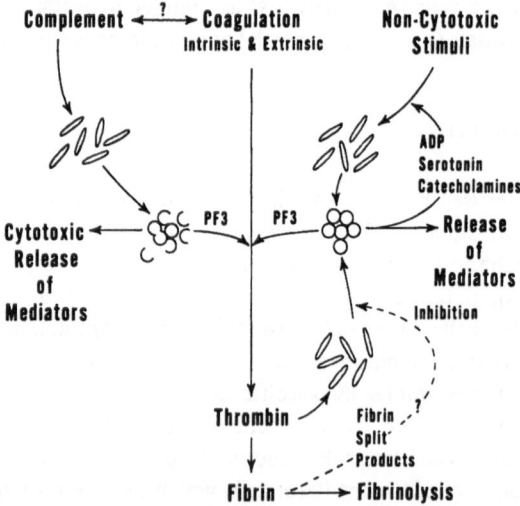

Fig. 2. Some interaction between the complement, coagulation, and fibrinolytic systems with stimulated or nonstimulated platelets to induce, enhance, or control release of platelet mediators. The platelets are depicted as discoid when normal and as round and aggregated when stimulated or lysed. Broken arrow represents inhibition.

3.1. Platelet Mediators

Two types of granules are predominant in platelets (see White, 1971). The "dense bodies" have been shown to contain the vasoactive amines of the platelets (serotonin in most species, histamine and serotonin in the rabbit) probably complexed ionically to ATP. These granules may also contain catecholamines. Lysosomal enzymes are probably located in the so-called α-granule. Cationic substances which induce vascular permeability have been detected (Mustard and Packham, 1970), and platelets also synthesize prostaglandins (Vane, 1971). Thus a wealth of potential mediators are associated with these highly reactive cells.

3.2. Morphology of the Release Reaction

In noncytotoxic release, the contents of the dense bodies are rapidly liberated—probably by discharge of the granule into the canalicular system (White and Estensen, 1972) or by exocytosis (Hobbs and Cliff, 1973). Preliminary evidence suggests that, as with mast cells, contact of the granule with cations from the extracellular fluid leads to dissolution of the granule and release of its contents (Uvnäs, 1971). Accompanying release (and aggregation), the platelets develop an irregular shape, a network of microtubules containing the platelet organelles apparently migrates toward the center of the cell, and the canalicular system disappears (Fig. 3) (White, 1971). These processes may be associated with contraction, and it is possible that this serves to extrude the contents of the canalicular system. However, the contraction is also related to other activities of platelets such as clot retraction. Moreover, contractile microfilaments may serve to bring granules and the canalicular system together or to open a channel between them.

3.3. Stimuli Inducing the Noncytotoxic Platelet Release Reactions

A wide variety of different stimuli may cause the platelet release reaction and/or aggregation. These include both soluble and particulate materials, low molecular weight inducers, and proteolytic enzymes (Mustard and Packham, 1970; Becker and Henson, 1973).

3.3.1. Collagen. Platelets adhere closely to collagen fibers, swell, and undergo the release reaction. Although of great potential importance in inflammatory processes, the nature of this reaction with collagen remains speculative (Puett *et al.*, 1973).

3.3.2. Thrombin. Thrombin and trypsin, but not chymotrypsin, directly

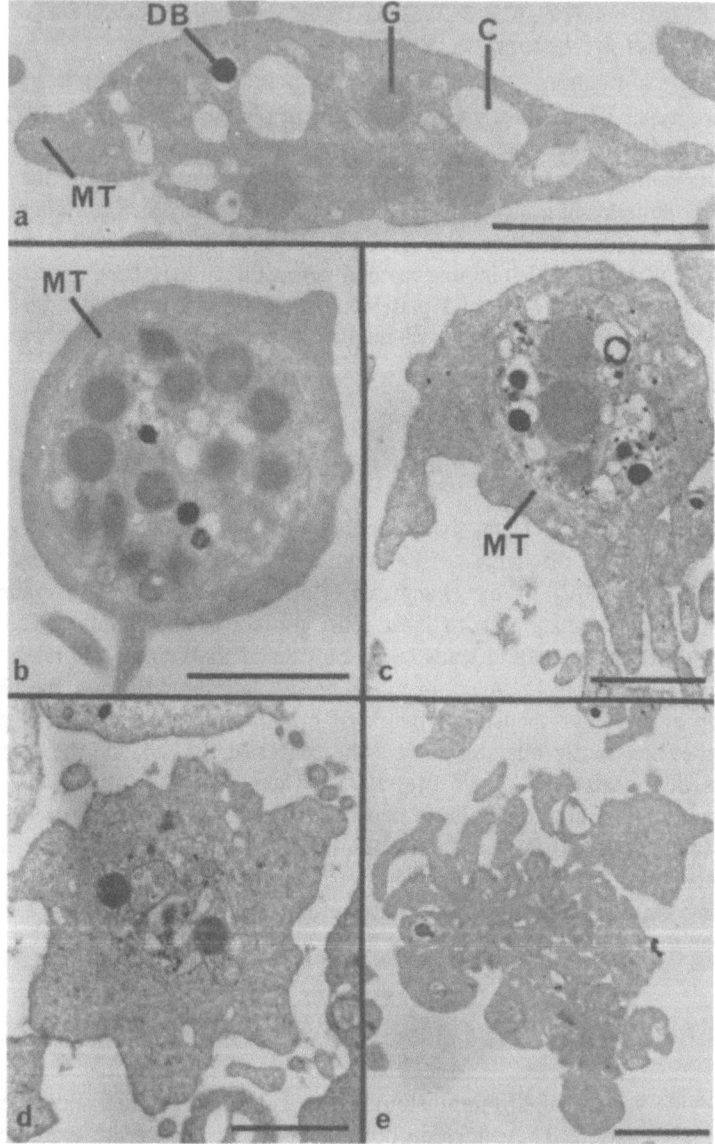

Fig. 3. Platelets. (a) Normal rabbit platelet showing the discoid shape, marginal bundles of microtubules (MT), dense bodies (DB), α-granules (G), and canalicular system (C). (b) Normal platelet sectioned at right angles to (a); the same features are present. (c,d,e) Progressive changes in platelets undergoing the release reaction, here stimulated by antiplatelet antibody. The ring of microtubules appears to move toward the center, enclosing the organelles, which eventually disappear (e).

stimulate noncytotoxic release of granule-associated constituents from platelets (Mustard and Packham, 1970). In high concentration, however, thrombin may also have an increasingly cytotoxic effect (Sneddon, 1972).

3.3.3. ADP. ADP is primarily an inducer of platelet aggregation (see below). However, in higher concentration it can initiate a release reaction from human platelets, which like the other release reactions liberates more ADP and is inhibited by, for example, aspirin (Zucker and Petersen, 1968).

3.3.4. Immunological Releasing Agents. In a discussion of immunological reactions of platelets, an important species distinction must be considered (see Becker and Henson, 1973). Mammalian platelets fall into two groups, on the basis of receptors for C3b. Rabbit, mouse, guinea pig, rat, dog, cat, and horse platelets have these receptors and undergo immune adherence. However, rabbit platelets (which have been the most extensively studied) do not readily react with aggregated immunoglobulin or directly with immune complexes. They appear to lack an immunoglobulin (Fc piece) receptor.

In contrast, human, baboon, pig, sheep, and ox platelets do not have a C3 receptor, and do not exhibit immune adherence. Human platelets do react directly with the Fc pieces of immunoglobulins G (all four subclasses). The immunoglobulin must be aggregated, in a complex, or adherent to particles or surfaces and induces a potent release reaction. Complement components in fact inhibit the reaction, probably by covering up the Fc piece (Pfueller and Lüscher, 1972; Henson and Spiegelberg, 1973).

The reaction of rabbit platelets with bound C3b by the C3 immune adherence site induces a release reaction. The release is markedly augmented by the presence of small numbers of neutrophils, providing an example of potentially important synergistic reactions between platelets and other cell types. However, the presence of later-acting complement components including C6 causes a cytotoxic reaction as well (see below).

Another immunological reaction involves the binding of antiplatelet antibody to rabbit (Henson, 1970) or human (Mueller-Eckhardt and Lüscher, 1968) platelets. In the absence of complement, a release reaction (and agglutination) results. This stimulation requires the antibody to be divalent.

3.3.5. Platelet-Activating Factors from Basophils or Mast Cells. Stimulated rabbit (and probably human) basophils release a low molecular weight activator which induces a release reaction in rabbit platelets (Henson and Benveniste, 1971). The nature of this platelet-activating factor (PAF) is unknown. It is liberated from the basophils along with the histamine which is released during their secretory reaction. There is also preliminary evidence for the release of a similar substance from rabbit mast cells (T. Kravis and P. M. Henson, unpublished observations). Since such PAFs are released during allergic reactions or following anaphylatoxin generation (Fig. 4), these interconnected release reactions represent important sources of inflammatory mediators.

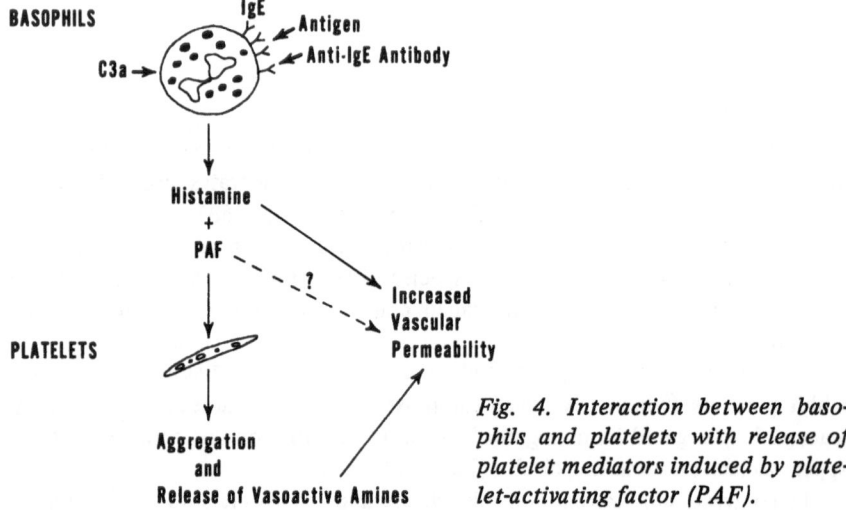

Fig. 4. Interaction between basophils and platelets with release of
platelet mediators induced by platelet-activating factor (PAF).

3.4. Mechanisms of Noncytotoxic Release from Platelets

The platelet is proving a useful cell for probing the mechanism of mediator secretion. Of additional interest is the close similarity between the processes involved in release and those involved in aggregation (Becker and Henson, 1973).

3.4.1. Serine Esterases and Platelet Activation. Serine esterase inhibitors or substrates prevent the release reaction. Secretion of serotonin from rabbit platelets induced by collagen, PAF, C3, and antiplatelet antibody is prevented by DFP but only if it is present during the reaction (Henson *et al.*, 1973). This suggests that the stimuli activate a precursor esterase (see Section 2.4.1.). Activity–structure inhibition profiles with different phosphonate inhibitors have provided circumstantial evidence that each stimulus activates a different pro-esterase (P. M. Henson and E. L. Becker, unpublished observations). It has been suggested that this activation represents the initial trigger to the cell and that thrombin and trypsin either bypass such platelet esterases and act directly (since they are themselves serine esterases) on the same substrates in the cell or in fact activate the proesterases (Becker and Henson, 1973).

3.4.2. Calcium Release requires Ca^{2+} in the medium, except for a few examples involving human platelets where, as evidenced by a measurable efflux of Ca^{2+}, internal sources of Ca^{2+} may be mobilized.

3.4.3. Cyclic AMP and Catecholamines. Increasing the platelet cAMP (e.g., by stimulation of adenylate cyclase with PGE_1, or by inhibition of phosphodiesterase, or by addition of cAMP itself) inhibits release. Decreasing cAMP (e.g., by α-adrenergic stimulation) enhances release (see Salzman, 1972; Becker and

Henson, 1973). During or preceding the release reaction, a temporary drop in intracellular cAMP has been noted with most of the stimuli. Despite the problems and caveats mentioned in Section 2.4.3., one possible mode of action for cAMP may be suggested. The stimuli induce a series of biochemical events in the platelets leading to release and, simultaneously, reduce cAMP levels (by inhibiting the adenylate cyclase or by some other mechanism) enough to permit these processes to proceed. The drop in cAMP is temporary, and as the level returns to normal the release reaction is halted. cAMP changes would thus act to control the reaction (Fig. 1).

3.4.4. Microtubules and Contractile Proteins (Thrombosthenin). Microtubules and contractile proteins are both of importance to the release reaction. For example, colchicine inhibits, and induces marked shape changes, but cytochalasin B may have variable effects (Becker and Henson, 1973; White and Estensen, 1972).

3.4.5. Order of Interaction. The suggested esterase activation precedes the requirement for Ca^{2+}, energy, and the step modulated by cAMP (Henson *et al.,* 1973).

3.5. Cytotoxic Reactions of Platelets

Cytotoxic reactions involving platelets also contribute to the release of mediators. Many materials including high concentrations of thrombin can induce lysis of platelets *in vitro.* However, *in vivo* it is probably the immunological reactions which have most relevance in this respect. Thrombocytopenia may result from lysis of platelets. However, increased clearance or turnover may also result from noncytotoxic reactions.

3.5.1. Immune Complexes and Complement. It is important again to distinguish between species in discussing the cytotoxic reactions. Incubation of immune complexes in antibody excess in *rabbit* platelet-rich plasma leads to a marked release of platelet constituents. This system has been extensively investigated (see Becker and Henson, 1973; Osler and Siraganian, 1972). It is now clear that a cytotoxic reaction results, that it involves complement, and that most platelet constituents, including membrane associated-coagulation factors, are liberated. The mechanism appears to be that of an "innocent bystander" reaction. The immune complexes bind C3 by the conventional or the alternate pathways of complement activation. They adhere to the C3 receptor of rabbit platelets. Meanwhile, they are still activating complement components. The C567 thus activated transfers to the platelet membrane and in the presence of C8 and C9 induces lysis of the platelets (Fig. 5). There is now much accumulated evidence for this hypothesis, and some of the most compelling comes from the demonstration that in plasma from rabbits deficient in C6 immune complexes and

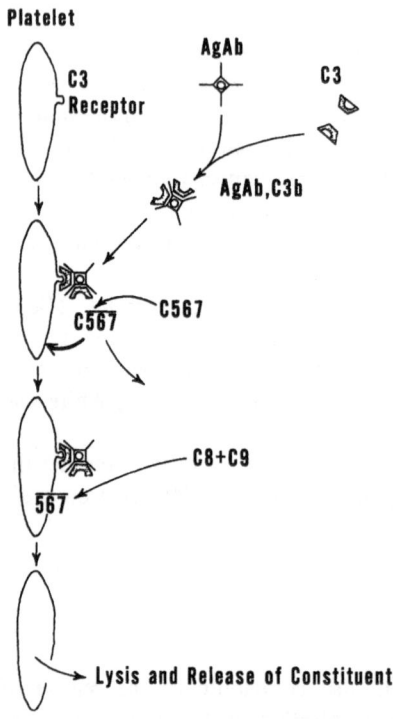

Platelet

Fig. 5. The "innocent bystander" complement-dependent cytotoxic release mechanism of rabbit platelets.

platelets interact without lysis (Henson, 1970). The lytic reaction returns if C6 is restored. In the absence of C3, however, no interaction occurs at all.

3.5.2. *Antibody and Complement.* Antibody to rabbit platelets in the *presence* of complement induces a similar cytotoxic release of constituents (Henson, 1970*a,b*). This is directly comparable mechanistically and observationally with the "innocent bystander" phenomenon described above. Here, however, the complement-fixing system (antibody) is directly reacting with the platelet membrane.

3.5.3. *Endotoxin.* An extensive literature on the effect of endotoxins on rabbit platelets (see DesPrez and Marney, 1971; Becker and Henson, 1973; Osler and Siraganian, 1972) suggests a very similar mechanism to that described for immune complexes. Endotoxin activates complement and causes lysis of rabbit platelets by a process involving complement components, including C6. It can be postulated again that C3 immune adherence brings endotoxin and platelets together (Spielvogel, 1967), allowing C$\overline{567}$ transfer to the platelets. Alternatively or indeed in addition, endotoxin may react directly with platelets, only later activating complement. However, there is little evidence that, if this be the case, it is not due to binding of endotoxin to adsorbed plasma protein on the platelets.

3.5.4. Human Platelets. Endotoxins do not induce release from human platelets (Nagayama *et al.,* 1971), which may reflect the lack of C3 receptors. Heterologous antibody to human platelets can cause a release reaction and, in the presence of complement, lysis of the platelets. However, the effect of factors (antibody?) present in the serum of some patients with idiopathic thrombocytopenic purpura (ITP) is less clear; this is also the case for the drug-induced, immunological thrombocytopenias (Shulman *et al.,* 1964). Recently, the hemorrhagic shock syndrome associated with dengue fever has gained prominence. Complement is consumed and there is a marked thrombocytopenia (Bokisch *et al.,* 1973). Virus–platelet or virus–antibody–platelet interaction may account for the platelet changes, but it is not known whether this is a complement-dependent lytic reaction or whether the aggregation and/or release is sufficient without any intervention of the complement system.

3.6. In Vivo Release from Platelets

Platelets are gaining increasing prominence as possible sources of inflammatory mediators *in vivo.* Recent evidence has suggested, for example, that IgE–antigen–basophil interactions in anaphylaxis can lead to platelet release *in vivo,* probably through the action of PAF (Halonen *et al.,* 1973). Endotoxin in rabbits also cuases thrombocytopenia and *in vivo* release from platelets (Brown and Lachmann, 1973). Immune complexes which form in the blood of rabbits induce the binding of platelets, with subsequent release of constituents and eventual thrombocytopenia (Movat *et al.,* 1968). This is abrogated in animals depleted of C3 (P. M. Henson and C. G. Cochrane, unpublished observations). Neutrophils may also be involved in such reactions, possibly providing additional stimuli to the platelets. Local formation of immune complexes in blood vessel walls (Arthus reaction) results in platelet accumulation, though their absolute requirement for the injury is controversial (Kravis and Henson, 1974). *In vivo* exocytosis from platelets has also been seen (Hobbs and Cliff, 1973).

The intimate interactions between platelets and the coagulation and complement systems (as is true of interactions between platelets and leukocytes) mean that activation of one or both often results in platelet release. Moreover, since many plasma proteins may interact in or on the platelet surface and platelets themselves provide phospholipid (factor 3) for the coagulation process, the platelet surface may provide an important site for action and interaction of both these systems. Involvement of platelets in coagulation results in liberation of many platelet constituents and mediators (Mustard and Packham, 1970). Damage to blood vessels also leads to platelet involvement, again with mediator release as part of the process. In addition, it should be emphasized that platelets have other functions such as involvement in blood vessel integrity and thrombosis (see Johnson, 1971).

4. MAST CELLS

The experimental work on the release of mediators from mast cells falls into two categories (see Becker and Henson, 1973). Isolated mast cells from the peritoneal cavity of the mouse and rat have provided important information as to mechanisms of release. Extensive investigation has also been directed toward release of mediators from perfused or chopped lung. Although there is good evidence that the mediators come from tissue mast cells, these represent but a very small proportion of the total number of cells present.

4.1. Mast Cell Mediators

Of prime importance is histamine, located in the characteristic dense granules of this cell, probably bound ionically to heparin. The effect of the heparin as a mediator is unknown. Mast cells from some species also contain 5-hydroxytryptamine (serotonin). Slow-reacting substance of anaphylaxis (SRS-A) probably also comes from the mast cell, as does the eosinophil chemotactic factor of anaphylaxis (ECFA) (Kay *et al.*, 1971). This last material may be important in explaining the accumulations of eosinophils often seen in allergic reactions.

4.2. Morphology of the Release from Mast Cells

The morphological events involved in release from isolated rat peritoneal mast cells are depicted in Fig. 6. There is a perigranular membrane fusion (see Lagunoff, 1973) and changes in the apparent granule density. It has been suggested that exposure of granules to cations in the external fluid leads to exchange for the electrostatic binding sites for histamine, resulting in solubilization and release of the histamine (see Uvnäs, 1971; Lagunoff, 1972). This could occur independently of granule extrusion, as long as there is fusion (leading to an opening) between granule membrane and external membrane. While this general mechanism seems to be true for rat and mouse peritoneal mast cells, those from the guinea pig may behave differently (see also Section 5.2).

4.3. Stimuli Inducing Release from Mast Cells

4.3.1. Homocytotropic Antibody. Immunoglobulin E binds to the surface of mast cells and triggers the release reaction when it reacts with specific antigen (see Becker and Henson, 1973). Antibody directed against IgE will also induce release. More weakly bound homocytotropic antibody (e.g., rat IgGa) is effec-

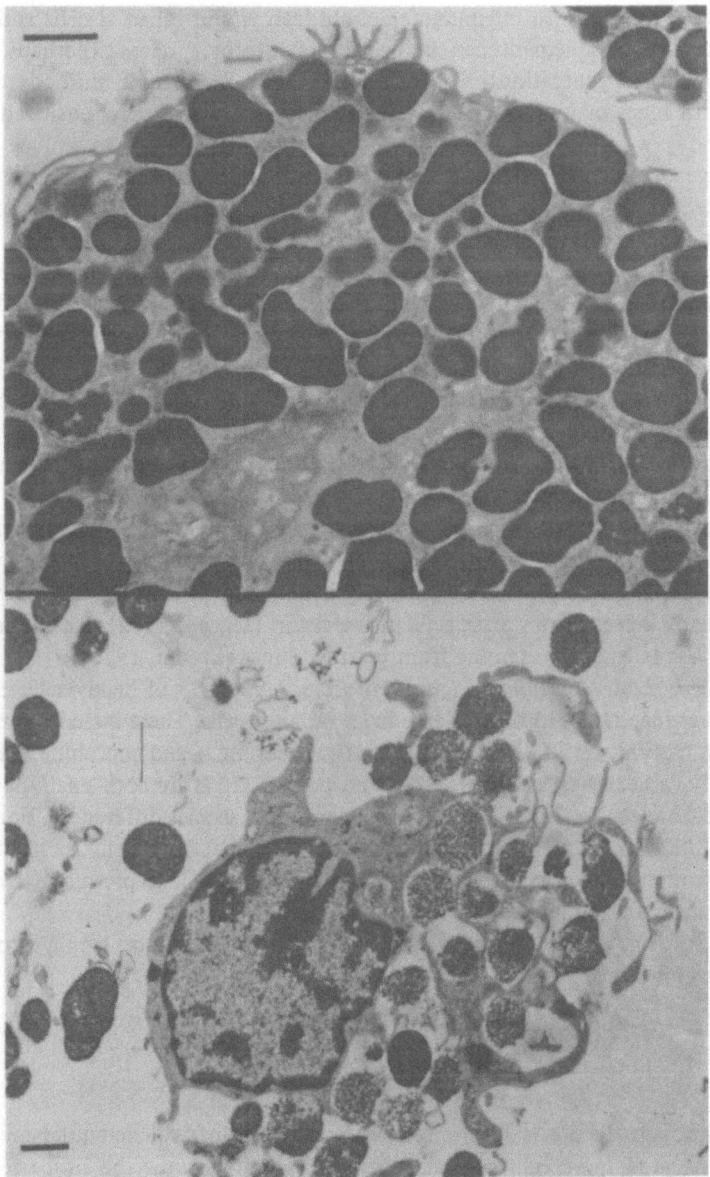

Fig. 6. Electron micrograph of rat peritoneal mast cells undergoing release. Top: Normal mast cell. Bottom: After interaction with anaphylatoxin. Note the intact cytoplasm and the partially disintegrating granules both extended from the cell and within intracytoplasmic spaces. Photographs courtesy of C. G. Cochrane.

tive, too. Antibody to rat immunoglobulin can trigger rat mast cells and in the presence of complement can induce a noncytotoxic release (perhaps due to anaphylatoxin generation). The reactions of homocytotropic antibody also occur with lungs or lung fragments. The tissues may be passively sensitized by the antibody, washed, and subsequently reacted with antigen to induce release (Orange *et al.*, 1971). In addition, perfusion of whole guinea pig lung with soluble immune complexes induces complement-independent release of histamine and mast cell degranulation (Broder, 1969).

4.3.2. Neutrophil Cationic Protein. Four small cationic proteins may be isolated from rabbit neutrophil granules, each of which increases vascular permeability on injection into the skin. One of them acts by inducing noncytotoxic release of amines from mast cells (Ranadive and Cochrane, 1971). The others do not, though they have very similar amino acid compositions. Since the cationic protein is actively released from neutrophils (Henson, 1971*a*; Hawkins and Peeters, 1971), the cell-to-cell cooperative effect may be important in generating more inflammatory mediators.

4.3.3. Anaphylatoxins. The small cationic fragments cleaved from the complement components C3 and C5 (C3a and C5a) induce release of histamine from mast cells. Both contract the guinea pig ileum, though this may only in part be caused by release from mast cells in the ileum (Jensen, 1972). Anaphylatoxins also cause release of histamine from perfused lungs (Broder, 1970).

4.3.4. Low Molecular Weight Activators. A variety of highly selective activators induce noncytotoxic release from rat mast cells. These include compound 48/80, polymyxin B, ATP, melittin, *d*-tubocurarine, and morphine. The first three have been best studied. 48/80 and polymyxin B are both small, positively charged molecules. However, there are significant species differences. For example, 48/80 is a highly potent activator of rat mast cells but has no such action on cells from the mouse (see Becker and Henson, 1973). It produces a variable bluing reaction in rabbit skin.

4.3.5. Enzymes. Chymotrypsin, but not trypsin, induces noncytotoxic release from rat mast cells.

4.4. Mechanisms of Release from Mast Cells

Although there are differences between release of granule-bound mediators from isolated mast cells and that from tissue fragments, the processes seem similar enough to consider together. Release by the abovementioned activators is noncytotoxic; cytoplasmic enzymes and nucleotides are not released (Johnson and Moran, 1969).

4.4.1. Serine Esterases. Release from rat mast cells by neutrophilic cationic protein or immunological stimuli is inhibited by DFP and phosphonate inhibitors (see Becker and Henson, 1973). This occurs only when the inhibitor is present during the reaction, which suggests that a serine esterase is activated by the stimulus–cell interaction, and is required for the release. This apparent requirement for serine esterase activation also applies to release from guinea pig and human lung fragments. Interestingly, the esterases (probably chymotrypsin-like) in the two systems are different (Becker and Austen, 1966), although with three different stimuli on isolated rat mast cells they appear to be the same. As mentioned, chymotrypsin itself induces release from mast cells, raising the possibility that it may act on the same substrate in the cell as the putative esterase or indeed may itself activate the esterase (see Section 2.4.1.).

4.4.2. Cations. The requirement for calcium in the medium is variable for release from rat peritoneal mast cells. As emphasized for platelets, however, this variability does not preclude the requirement for Ca^{2+}, which may be supplied from intracellular sources, although an accumulation of Ca^{2+} has been demonstrated during ATP-induced release (Dahlquist *et al.*, 1973). Release can in fact be induced by calcium ionophores, which permit the selective cellular accumulation of Ca^{2+} (Foreman *et al.*, 1973). For release from human lung fragments, Ca^{2+} appears to be required at two stages of the process (Section 4.4.5).

4.4.3. Cyclic Nucleotides. The effect of agents which increase cAMP have been studied on release from human lung fragments. Such agents (PGE_1, theophylline, β-adrenergic stimuli) inhibit the release of histamine and SRS-A. By contrast, α-adrenergic stimulation causes increased release (Orange *et al.*, 1971). This suggests that decreased cAMP levels might enhance the release. To confirm this it would be necessary to measure such a decrease in the mast cells, which in view of their low density in the tissues is not possible. Isoproterenol (β-agonist) does certainly increase cAMP levels in the tissue as a whole, and epinephrine plus propranolol does decrease them (Kaliner *et al.*, 1971), but this says little about the mast cells themselves. Nor is there any indication of cAMP changes in the normal secretory process. Similarly, stimulators of adenyl cyclase or inhibitors of phosphodiesterase prevent release from peritoneal mast cells, though the effects of catecholamines may be less clear than for the lung tissues (Stechschulte and Austen, 1973).

Cholinergic stimuli enhance release from lung fragments, and this has been suggested to result from stimulation of increased cGMP (Kaliner *et al.*, 1972). This would imply an antagonistic effect between cAMP and cGMP which might serve to control the release process. While there is as yet little evidence in this system to confirm or define such a controlling mechanism, it does present an intriguing possibility which is being examined in a number of different cells.

4.4.4. Microtubules and Contractile Proteins. Mast cells contain microtubules, and disruption of these, for example, by colchicine, prevents the release of histamine (Padawer, 1969). Deuterium oxide enhances release and increases microtubule aggregation (Gillespie *et al.*, 1968). These data suggest an as yet undefined role for microtubules in the release (degranulation) process. There is no clear evidence for an involvement of microfilaments in release from mast cells, although an inhibitory action of cytochalasin B has been reported (Orr *et al.*, 1972).

4.4.5. Order of Interaction. As was originally shown by Ranadive and Cochrane (1971), the release from rat mast cells can be divided into stages. Interaction with neutrophilic cationic protein in the presence of reversible inhibitors leads to an "activated" state in which the cells are poised, ready to continue the release process as soon as the inhibition is reversed, even if the activator has meanwhile been removed. By use of such techniques, the events required for the release reaction can be sequenced. Thus esterase activation occurs before the temperature-sensitive event, which itself occurs before divalent cations are required. Similar experiments performed with antigen-induced release from passively sensitized human lung fragments have revealed two Ca^{2+}-requiring steps (Kaliner and Austen, 1973). One occurs very early, perhaps preceding the esterase activation. It has been suggested that the early Ca^{2+} requirement may indicate a proesterase in the mast cell which requires Ca^{2+} for its function and/or activiation by IgE and antigen. Kaliner *et al.* (1973) have pointed out the analogy between the activation of C1 by IgG and that by antigen, which also requires Ca^{2+}. The second requirement for Ca^{2+} follows esterase activation, energy requirement, and perhaps cAMP modulation.

4.4.6. Inhibitors. In addition to those inhibitors mentioned above, disodium chromoglycate inhibits release from mast cells (Kusner *et al.*, 1972) and is proving a useful specific therapeutic agent. *In vivo*, sympathomimetic amines may play a very important controlling and inhibitory role in mediator release from mast cells, and such drugs are commonly used therapeutically. Prostaglandins released from the lung may also act as feedback controls of release.

4.5. Cytotoxic Reactions of Mast Cells

Cytotoxic reactions are known *in vitro* (anti-mast-cell antibody in the presence of complement, Valentine *et al.*, 1967), but their *in vivo* occurrence or significance is unknown.

4.6 In Vivo Release From Mast Cells

There is extensive indirect evidence for mast cell release *in vivo* (see Keller, 1966). This varies from morphological evidence of degranulation in passive cutaneous anaphylactic reactions (Bauer *et al.*, 1972) to the protective effects of inhibitors of the release process.

5. BASOPHILS

The basophil has proved a useful model for developing an understanding of cellular release processes and may provide an important source of mediators in some forms of inflammatory injury (Osler *et al.,* 1968). Most information has come from study of basophils from human and rabbit blood, although pure populations of these cells are not satisfactorily obtainable.

5.1. Basophil Mediators

Basophils contain electron-dense, membrane-bound granules which are morphologically different from those of mast cells. The prime mediator released from basophils is histamine, and in most species (rabbit excepted) they provide the main source of blood histamine. Rabbit (and probably human) basophils also liberate a platelet-activating factor (Benveniste *et al.,* 1973).

5.2. Morphology of the Release

Little is known of the release process. As observed in the electron microscope, the granules of rabbit basophils appear to become increasingly disrupted *in situ* (Fig. 7) but are not extruded. In contrast, exocytosis of granules can occur in tumor rejection and in "cutaneous basophil hypersensitivity" in guinea pigs (Dvorak *et al.,* 1973). It is clearly possible, though not proven, that the two-stage mechanism attributed to mast cells and perhaps platelets, i.e., opening (by an unknown process) of the granule contents to the outside followed by exchange solubilization of the ionically bound mediators, is also operative in basophils. On the other hand, the cells behave in some respects like other granulocytes (see Section 6). After release, basophils lose their metachromatically staining granules.

5.3. Stimuli Inducing Basophil Release

The stimulus most studied has been that of homocytotropic antibody (IgE) on the cell reacting with antigen or with anti-IgE antibody. The IgE molecules bind to surface receptors by virtue of their Fc regions. On reaction with anti-IgE, a temperature-dependent aggregation of IgE molecules into "patches" on the surface is seen (Sullivan *et al.,* 1971), although whether this is required for cell stimulation is unknown.

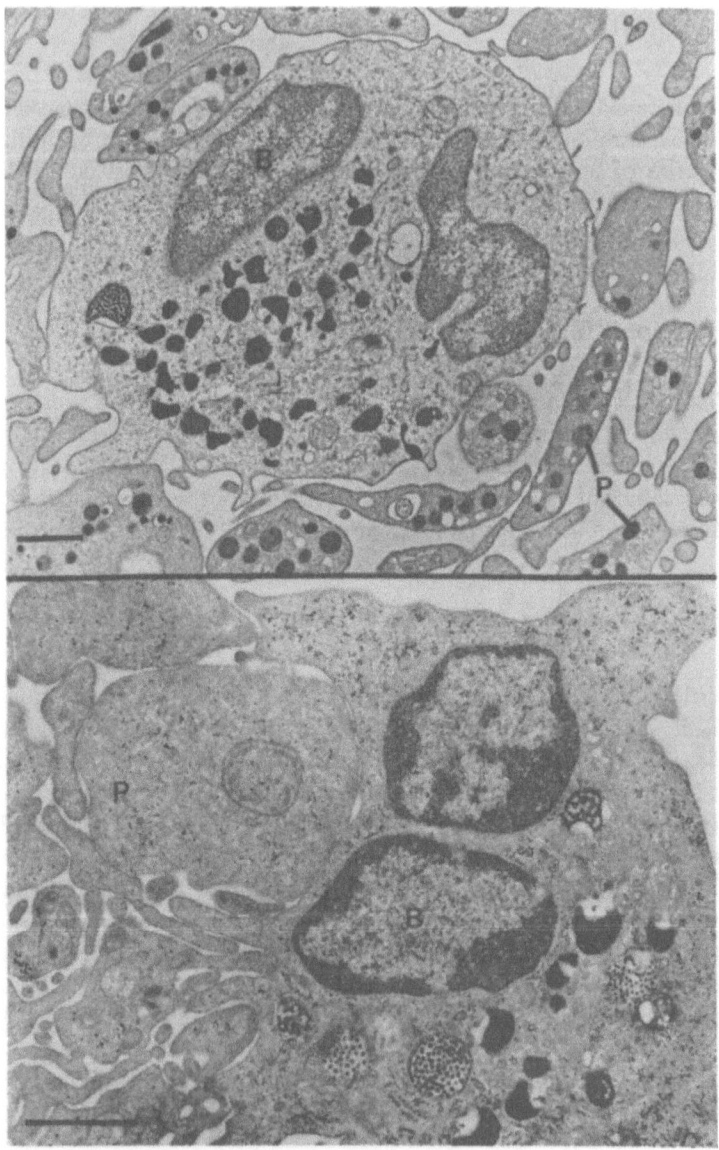

Fig. 7. The release process in rabbit basophils. Top: Normal circulating basophil from a sensitized rabbit surrounded by platelets (P). Bottom: Basophil during release (stimulated by antigen). The granules exhibit various degrees of morphological disintegration *in situ*. Note that the platelets have also undergone a release reaction (see Fig. 4). From Benveniste *et al.* (1973).

5.4. Mechanisms of Release from Basophils

5.4.1. Serine Esterases. A requirement for activation of serine esterases has not been clearly demonstrated in basophils (see Becker and Henson, 1973).

5.4.2. Cations. Ca^{2+} is required in the medium for release.

5.4.3. Cyclic Nucleotides. Lichtenstein and Margolis (1968) showed that agents which increase cAMP inhibit release of histamine from basophils. These include PGE_1, β-adrenergic agents, and phosphodiesterase inhibitors. Cholera enterotoxin produces a delayed but prolonged stimulation of adenylate cyclase which correlates well with inhibition of release (Bourne *et al.*, 1973). Histamine itself has recently been shown to inhibit the release of histamine (Lichtenstein and Gillespie, 1973) by virtue of the presence of H_2-receptors on the basophils, possibly because of its ability to increase adenyl cyclase activity. While it has not been possible to examine cAMP changes in the basophil alone, studies on whole leukocyte populations have revealed good correlation between cAMP levels and the inhibitory effect of increased cAMP on release (Bourne *et al.*, 1972).

5.4.4. Microtubules and Microfilaments. Colchicine inhibits release, while D_2O enhances it. Cytochalasin B also enhances the release (Gillespie and Lichtenstein, 1972). These preliminary findings suggest that the microtubules and microfilaments may be in some way involved.

5.4.5. Order of Interaction. Order of interaction has been studied (Lichtenstein, 1971) by experiments similar to those described above for platelets and mast cells. cAMP modulation of release occurs before the Ca^{2+} requirement, which itself precedes or accompanies steps requiring energy metabolism and microtubule function. Holding the "activated" but reversibly inhibited cells for increasing lengths of time results in "desensitization" or decay, as seen with platelets and mast cells.

6. NEUTROPHILS

Neutrophils exhibit a variety of activities which are intimately connected with the pathogenesis of inflammatory reactions. These include chemotaxis, phagocytosis (engulfment), degranulation and release of granule constituents, and, finally, increased metabolic processes, resulting in bactericidal activities and acid production.

Following phagocytosis of a particle, the neutrophil granules discharge their contents of lysosomal enzymes into the vacuoles. It is now apparent that during the process some of these lysosomal constituents gain access to the extracellular environment without lysis of the cell; i.e., the cells undergo a secretory reaction

(Weissmann *et al.,* 1971*a*; Becker and Henson, 1973). If, *in vitro* or *in vivo,* the neutrophil reacts with potentially phagocytosable material (e.g., aggregated immunoglobulin) bound to a surface too extensive to be taken into the cell, it adheres to the surface and "degranulates" directly to the outside of the cell, i.e., a process of exocytosis (Hawkins, 1971; Henson, 1971*a,b*).

6.1. Neutrophil Mediators

Neutrophil mediators will be discussed in Chapter 2. Included among the important tissue-damaging constituents are factors which may act as mediators by influencing other cells or tissues (see Becker and Henson, 1973). Examples include the cationic protein which induces release from mast cells, factors which may induce release from platelets, factors in turn chemotactic for more neutrophils, factors which may enhance release from basophils, and endogenous pyrogen which induces increased body temperature. Pyrogen appears not to be prepackaged in the granules but may be synthesized *de novo* following stimulation of the cell (Bodel, 1970). Its mechanism of secretion is unknown. Indirect evidence suggests that SRS-A production in the rat peritoneal cavity may involve neutrophils. Procoagulant activity has been attributed to neutrophils, especially following interaction with endotoxin, and this has been shown to be primarily a tissue factor and to activate coagulation by the extrinsic pathway.

6.2. Morphology of Release from Neutrophils

6.2.1. Adherence, Phagocytosis, and Degranulation. The phagocytic process starts with adherence of neutrophils to the particles, which then become enclosed by the cell membrane. This eventually fuses to create a vacuole. Neutrophil granules are then liberated into the vacuoles as a result of fusion between the granule membrane and the vacuole membrane (Fig. 8). It should be emphasized that degranulation occurs only into vacuoles (or at membrane sites associated with adherence of particles), not at remote portions of the membrane. It is not known whether the granules are directed or moved toward the vacuole or whether they meet it by chance (see below).

6.2.2. Release During Phagocytosis. As depicted in Fig. 8, four related mechanisms have been demonstrated whereby granule contents, in the process of being discharged into vacuoles, may gain access to the outside of the cell (Weissmann *et al.,* 1972; Henson, 1973): (a) If the vacuole has not yet completely closed off (Fig. 9) or (b) if a preformed vacuole later opens to take in another particle, the granules may be liberated. (c) If two cells are involved in attempting to phagocytose a single particle, discharge of granules into the space between them in which the particle is enclosed may occur. (d) If the membranes

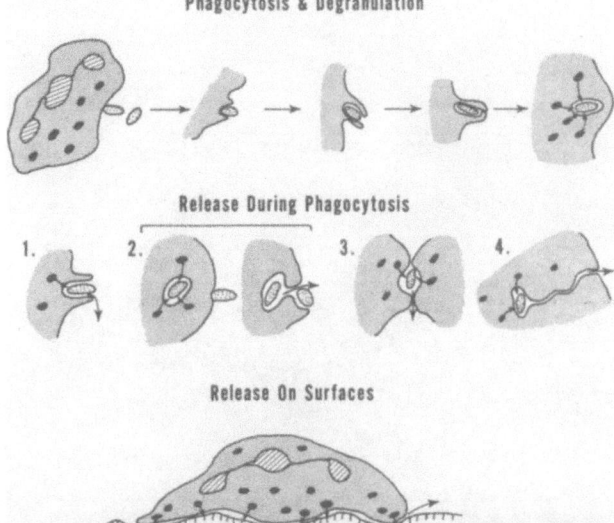

Phagocytosis & Degranulation

Release During Phagocytosis

Release On Surfaces

Fig. 8. Neutrophils. Diagrammatic representation of (top) secretion of granules into phagocytic vacuoles (degranulation), (middle) four different but related mechanisms of release to the outside of the cell during phagocytosis, and (bottom) release (exocytosis) from neutrophils on nonphagocytosable surfaces.

of the pseudopods enveloping the particle do not fuse, the vacuole may be connected to the outside of the cell by a narrow slit.

6.2.3. *Release on Nonphagocytosable Surfaces.* Activating substances attached to surfaces promote adherence of neutrophils and discharge of granules along the adherent cell membrane (Fig. 9). This exocytosis does not occur at portions of membrane not involved in adherence to the surface. Not all the granules are discharged, suggesting some control over granule movement and/or involvement of granules only with stimulated portions of the external membrane. Most of the granule contents are liberated into the medium. However, some, notably alkaline phosphatase, remain attached to the external membrane (Henson, 1971*a,b*). In both degranulation and exocytosis in rabbit neutrophils, the specific granules are released earlier than the azurophil granules.

6.3. Stimuli Inducing Neutrophil Release

Neutrophils have separate receptors for C3 and the Fc region of immunoglobulins G (all four subclasses) and immunoglobulins A (see Becker and Henson,

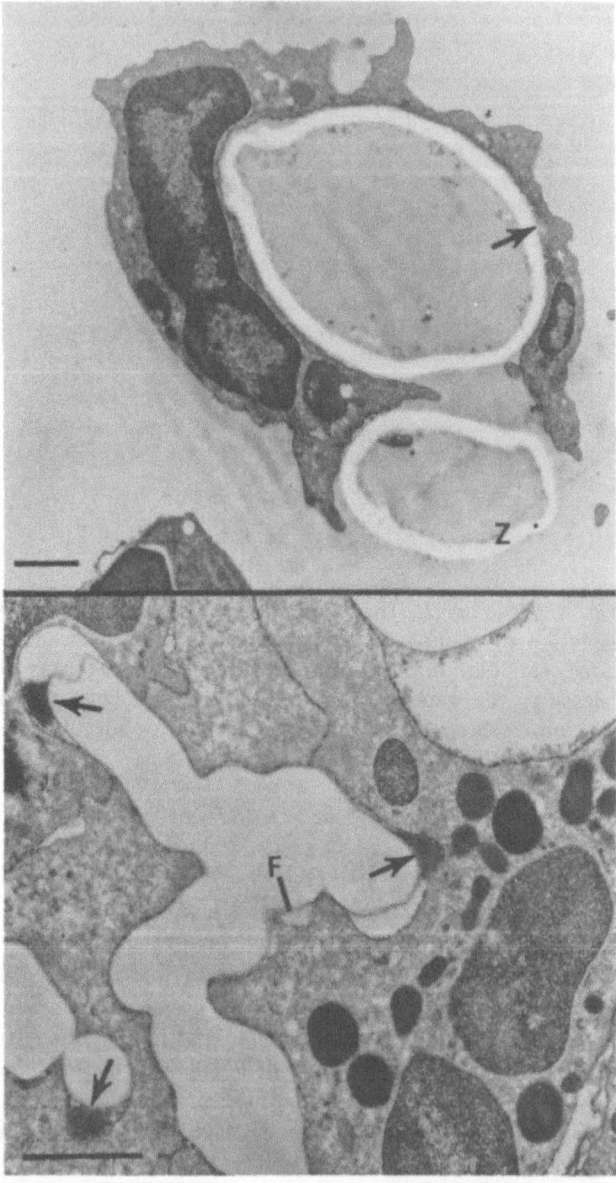

Fig. 9. Neutrophils. Top: Secretion of a neutrophil phagocytosing zymosan particles (Z) in which a granule (arrow) is
being liberated into a vacuole which is clearly open to the
outside. Bottom: Neutrophil on a filter (F) to which antigen and antibody are bound. Specific granules (arrows) are
being liberated along the filter surface (exocytosis). From
Henson (1971*b*).

1973). The first must be cleaved to expose the adherence site, which is on the C3b portion of the molecule. In order to activate the neutrophils, the immunoglobulins must be bound to antigen or aggregated. Both C3 and immunoglobulin promote phagocytosis and degranulation. They also stimulate increased glucose oxidation through the hexose monophosphate shunt (HMS). Other types of particles are phagocytosed by neutrophils, but this is usually inefficient in the absence of serum (which possibly supplies C3 or immunoglobulin). The release of granule constituents has been most studied using bacteria or zymosan particles in the presence of serum or those which have bound serum components.

A number of factors are known to be chemotactic to neutrophils, causing migration of the cells through a micropore filter. Such factors include C3a, C5a, $\overline{C567}$, a variety of denatured proteins, and a low molecular weight factor from bacterial cultures. It has recently been shown that these factors also stimulate release of granule enzymes if presented to neutrophils in the presence of a micropore filter or with cytochalasin B (Becker et al., 1974; Goldstein et al., 1973).

Requirement for a surface: To induce release of granule enzymes, it appears that the stimuli must be presented to the neutrophil on an insoluble particle or surface. This requirement is also true for phagocytosis and partially so for metabolic stimulation. Chemotaxis too is probably a surface phenomenon (Henson, unpublished observations). Mildly aggregated but soluble immunoglobulin does not induce neutrophils in suspension to release lysosomal enzymes, but if the immunoglobulin is attached to surfaces it is highly effective in stimulating exocytosis (Becker and Henson, 1973). While it is not known how the surface contributes to the reaction, one possibility is that stimuli presented in this manner aggregate receptors in the membrane more effectively. Some such localized deformation of the membrane may be required (a) to trigger membrane changes involved in movement and/or pseudopod formation and (b) to trigger membrane changes which allow granule membranes to fuse with the internal surface of the plasma membrane.

6.4. Mechanisms of Release from Neutrophils

While the following discussion will concentrate on release from neutrophils (and degranulation), the related processes of engulfment, HMP stimulation, and chemotaxis will also be mentioned.

6.4.1. Serine Esterases. DFP inhibits the release of granule enzymes and HMP stimulation. However, it is not yet clear whether a proesterase is activated by the stimulus or whether the DFP is acting on an enzyme which is already active (Henson, 1972). Chemotaxis does involve the activation of a neutrophil serine esterase for which low molecular weight synthetic substrates have been found (see Becker, 1972). Phagocytosis too may require activation of a serine esterase (Pearlman *et al.*, 1969).

6.4.2. Divalent Cations. The neutrophil activities require calcium. Rabbit neutrophils require Ca^{2+} in the medium, but human neutrophils may be able to mobilize an intracellular source (see Becker and Henson, 1972).

6.4.3. Cyclic Nucleotides. As with other mediator cells, PGE_1, theophylline, and high doses of cAMP increase intracellular cAMP in neutrophils and inhibit release (Weissmann *et al.*, 1971*a*; Bourne *et al.*, 1971; Zurier *et al.*, 1973*b*, 1974). Some difficulties have been encountered in considering a controlling or initiating role for cyclic AMP in degranulation or release from neutrophils (Henson, 1972; Hawkins, 1972*b*; Bourne *et al.*, 1973). In particular, this has been related to discrepant concentrations of agents required to increase cAMP and to inhibit release, and to the observation that cholera enterotoxin, which markedly increases cAMP, does not prevent release. This latter problem has been resolved by the finding that different preparations of enterotoxins differ in their biological effects (Zurier *et al.*, 1974). Epinephrine also appears to be a poor inhibitor, though it does increase cAMP in neutrophils (Scott, 1970). While it appears that cAMP *can* inhibit release, it is by no means clear that it does under natural circumstances. However, significant changes were observed in cAMP levels in purified neutrophils undergoing release (Zurier *et al.*, 1974).

Recently, a stimulating role for cGMP has been postulated, and an enhancing effect of this nucleotide, and of cholinergic agents, on release from neutrophils has been described (Ignarro, 1973; Zurier *et al.*, 1974). The two cyclic nucleotides therefore again seem to act in opposition to control the release process.

The picture is no less confusing for the role of the cyclic nucleotides in other neutrophil activities (see Becker and Henson, 1973). There is little evidence for any inhibition of phagocytosis by increases in endogenous cAMP, although exogenous cAMP clearly inhibits HMP stimulation (Weissmann *et al.*, 1971*b*; Cox and Karnovsky, 1973). The effect on chemotaxis seems varied and appears to suffer from many of the discrepancies seen for release. Again, a role for cAMP is neither proven nor excluded. Neither is there any indication whether cAMP may act directly as a messenger or as a control mechanism. A cAMP-dependent protein kinase has been described in neutrophils which was considered to be a mediator of cAMP inhibition of enzyme release by virtue of its potential phosphorylation of microtubules (Tsung and Weissmann, 1973). Recently, cGMP and agents which increase it in neutrophils have been shown to enhance chemotaxis, again demonstrating the opposing influences of the two nucleotides (Estensen *et al.*, 1973).

6.4.4. Energy Metabolism. Release and degranulation require energy metabolism, supplied in this cell by glycolysis. Glycolytic activity is also required for phagocytosis, chemotaxis, and hexose monophosphate pathway (HMP) stimulation. While HMP activity is increased by the stimuli and does provide additional ATP, it is not required for any of the other activities (Becker and Henson, 1973). Increased glycolysis, which also follows activation of neutrophils, probably provides the lactic acid which accumulates in the vacuoles. The release of vacuole contents may therefore contribute to the inflammatory process by lowering the pH.

6.4.5. *Microtubules.* Colchicine and related drugs have been reported to partially inhibit degranulation (Malawista, 1971) and to reduce release of lysosomal enzymes during phagocytosis (Zurier *et al.*, 1974; Weissmann *et al.*, 1972). In contrast, deuterium oxide (D_2O), which promotes microtubule disassembly, enhances enzyme release (Zurier *et al.*, 1974). Inhibition by colchicine of release from neutrophils on surfaces (Henson, 1972; Hawkins, 1972b) has been more difficult to demonstrate, although there are some reports of this (Zurier *et al.*, 1973b). The data suggest a partial involvement of microtubules in bringing or directing granules to their site of discharge (the vacuole). Neutrophils on surfaces are very spread out and only the granules nearest to the surface are released, so that less microtubular control or direction of the granules is required. During phagocytosis, however, degranulation is more extensive, requiring greater movement of granules within the cell. Microtubules may serve to maintain some shape to the cell, allowing or perhaps channeling movement of some of the distant granules to the vacuoles (which may or may not be open to the outside). Thus lack of microtubules would not completely prevent the process but could reduce its extent. An interesting and possibly related phenomenon is the observed link between a colchicine-binding protein associated with the neutrophil membrane and membrane particle movement such as may be involved in cell activation (Ukena and Berlin, 1972).

6.4.6. *Contractile Elements.* Neutrophils contain actinomyosinoid protein (Shibata *et al.*, 1972), and some stimuli have recently been shown to induce an expansion of the cell (Becker *et al.*, 1974). On the other hand, contraction is seen with glycerinated cells treated with ATP and Ca^{2+}. The connection between cell volume changes, microfilament function, and release of constituents is unclear. Cytochalasin B enhances exocytosis of granules from neutrophils (Zurier *et al.*, 1973a; Becker and Henson, 1973). The fungal agent prevents engulfment, and as a consequence the particles adhere to the neutrophil and the granules are discharged not into vacuoles (which are not formed) but to the outside (Zurier *et al.*, 1973a, 1974). The processes involved in uptake are prevented, but not apparently the changes in external membrane required for interaction with the granule membranes. Enhanced release is apparently due to increased movement of granules within the cytoplasm, perhaps resulting from disruption of peripheral, restraining microfilaments. This presumably allows more extensive interaction with the stimulated portion of the cell membrane (Henson and Oades, 1972; Allison *et al.*, 1971). Whether this is totally the result of disrupted microfilaments is not known since cytochalasin also inhibits glucose uptake into neutrophils (Zigmond and Hirsch, 1972) and may have other effects. Cytochalasin B exhibits a biphasic effect (high concentrations inhibit and low doses enhance) on both phagocytosis and chemotaxis.

6.4.7. Order of Interaction. It is not yet known in what order the above requirements are involved in the release process. It has been suggested that, as for platelets, esterase activation is an early step and that Ca^{2+} and ATP are required for the contractile processes which may be required. The possible controlling action of cAMP may be tied to the microtubule function (Zurier *et al.*, 1974) (see above), and this might explain the discrepant results obtained in attempting to show an absolute requirement for either system.

6.4.8. Inhibitors. Free immunoglobulin is an important inhibitor of the reaction of aggregated immunoglobulin or immune complexes with neutrophils; when present in the extracellular medium it acts as a competitive inhibitor for cell-surface receptors (Lay and Nussenzweig, 1968). However, if complement is fixed, this interacts with different receptors. Pharmacological and neuropharmacological agents may control release (and other neutrophil functions) as they do the other cell reactions. Once again, interplay between adrenergic and cholinergic stimulation is important. Prostaglandins also may contribute to control of release from neutrophils.

Of particular interest in this cell is an inhibitor of granule proteases which is found in the cytoplasm (Davies *et al.*, 1971). Its presence indicates the importance of secretion rather than cytotoxicity as a means of liberating active proteolytic mediators of inflammation.

6.5. Cytotoxic Reactions of Neutrophils

A number of agents induce a cytotoxic reaction which results in loss of granule and cytoplasmic enzymes. These reactions may include some of the processes involved in secretion.

6.5.1. Leukocidin. Woodin and his collaborators have extensively studied the effect of a staphyloccoccal product, leukocidin, on rabbit neutrophils (Woodin and Wieneke, 1970). The reaction is cytotoxic but also induces some selective release of granule enzymes; it requires Ca^{2+} and perhaps ATP, but does not need glycolysis. On treatment with small amounts of leukocidin, the cells round up and the granules exhibit Brownian movement. It was suggested that the granule membranes react with triphosphoinositide and Ca^{2+} in the cell membrane, and following a later exclusion of the Ca^{2+} (brought about by ATP), fuse with the cell membrane to allow discharge of granule contents. There is as yet little evidence for the occurrence of this process.

6.5.2. Streptolysin O, Vitamin A, Antineutrophil Antibody and Complement. Streptolysin O, vitamin A, and antineutrophil antibody and complement exhibit properties similar to those of leukocidin, inducing massive granule enzyme release in a reaction which requires Ca^{2+} but is in fact eventually cytotoxic (Woodin and Wieneke, 1970; Davies et al., 1973). Heterologous antineutrophil antibody and complement eventually induce total lysis of the cell. However, preceding cell lysis, granule enzymes seem to be selectively released (Hawkins, 1972a). This process is of interest since it resembles the release of lysosomal enzymes from bone rudiments incubated with antibody and complement, a process also mimicked by vitamin A (see Becker and Henson, 1973).

6.5.3. *Urate Crystals and Silica.* Urate crystals are avidly phagocytosed by neutrophils. The end result of this process is not selective granule release but a cytotoxic reaction. The phagocytosis is normal, but the crystals then react with the vacuole membrane, possibly by hydrogen bonding, and cause its disruption. Release of lysosomal enzymes from the vacuoles into the cytoplasm is then a cytotoxic process. However, the enzymes must first have gained access to the vacuoles, and this is presumably by the normal secretory degranulation process. This explains the inhibition of urate-induced extracellular release by PGE_1 and colchicine (Zurier et al., 1973b).

6.6. Release from Neutrophils In Vivo

Neutrophils are a constituent part of many inflammatory reactions. Depletion of these cells from the body by various means has been used to demonstrate their essential role in the tissue injury associated with acute inflammation. This is in large part assumed to result from the release of lysosomal proteases. *In vivo* phagocytosis can be seen histologically to include degranulation into vacuoles. Release to the outside has been shown indirectly, for example, by detecting specific neutrophil enzymes in the urine during neutrophil-dependent glomerular injury, and directly by histological observations (Henson, 1972; Schumaker and Agudelo, 1971) (Fig. 10). *In vivo* evidence of chemotaxis of neutrophils to sites of complement fixation has also been described.

7. MACROPHAGES

There is much less information available on the release of mediators from macrophages. The cells are highly phagocytic; within them are granules (primary lysosomes) which discharge their contents into phagocytic vacuoles to create the secondary lysosomes and which contain enzymes capable of acting as mediators of inflammation. In this respect, they exhibit properties similar to those de-

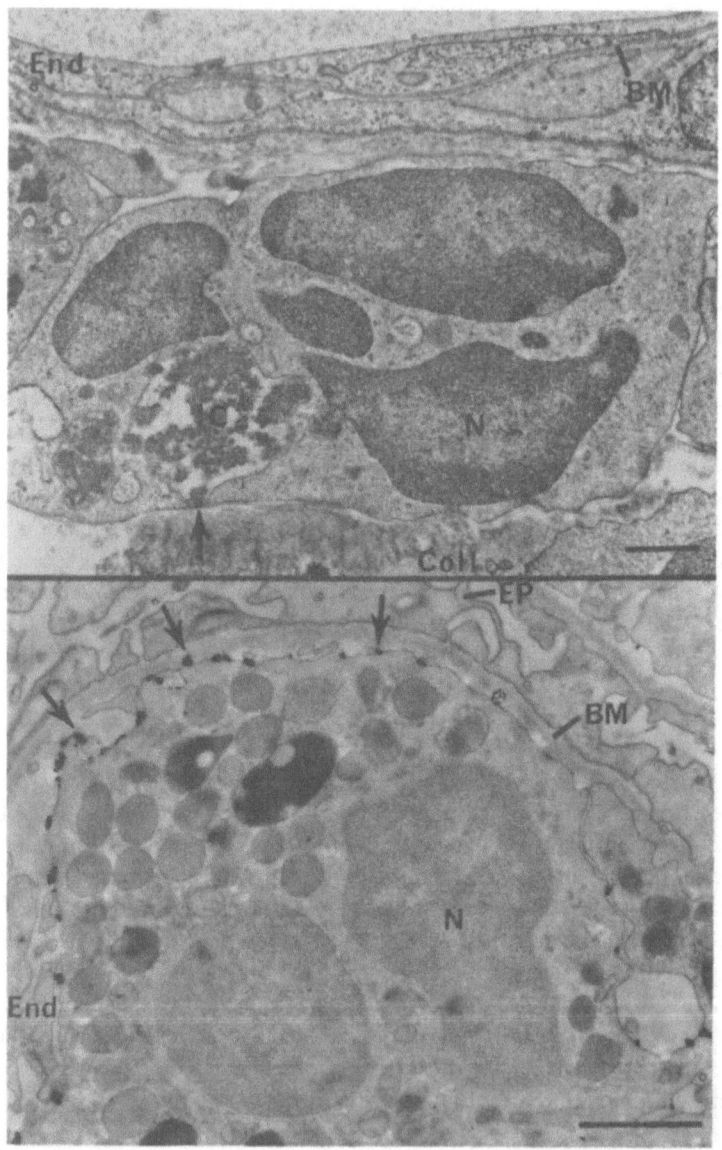

Fig. 10. Neutrophils in inflammatory reactions. Top: Neutrophil (N) outside a venule in an Arthus reaction in the rabbit bladder wall. End, Endothelial cells; BM, basement membrane; Coll, collagen fibers. Immune complexes (IC) may be seen in a vacuole which is open to the outside of the cell. Only a few granules are left in the cytoplasm. From Henson (1972). Bottom: Neutrophil along the basement membrane of a glomerular loop in the kidney of a rabbit undergoing nephrotoxic nephritis. The basement membrane (BM) has antibody and complement bound to it. EP, Epithelial cells; End, endothelial cells. The arrows point to the reaction product generated by the enzyme alkaline phosphatase which has been liberated from the neutrophil (it resides in the specific granules) and remains attached to the neutrophil plasma membrane. From Henson (1972).

scribed for neutrophils. However, they also undergo pinocytosis and have the additional property of synthesizing lysosomal enzymes following a variety of stimuli.

Recently, evidence has been obtained that during phagocytosis by macrophages granule enzymes may be released to the outside under conditions where cytoplasmic materials are retained (Weissmann *et al.*, 1971*a,b*). This release requires Ca^{2+} and has been reported to be prevented by colchicine and vinblastine, although at concentrations which inhibit uptake of the particles. This contrasts with the work of Allison *et al.* (1971), who showed no inhibition of uptake with colchicine, which nevertheless did prevent saltatory movements of the vacuoles. Cytochalasin B prevented phagocytosis but not micropinocytosis, and it enhanced granule enzyme release as it did in neutrophils (see Davies *et al.*, 1973). Release was inhibited by cAMP and cGMP. However, cyclic $2',3'$-AMP was also effective (Weissmann *et al.*, 1971*a,b*). The role of cyclic nucleotides thus requires further study.

The evidence is sparse as yet but does provide early indication that release from monocytes and macrophages may be very similar in mechanism to that seen in the other cells discussed, in particular to that from neutrophils.

8. MEDIATOR RELEASE AS A SECRETORY PHENOMENON

Striking similarities are apparent between the mechanisms of the release phenomena described above and secretory processes in general (see Becker and Henson, 1973). These secretory processes may vary as widely as release of acetylcholine from nerve endings to release of hormones and enzymes from the pancreas. Although morphological details vary, in many of these cases, as in the release of mediators, the product to be secreted is present in membrane-bound vesicles or granules and its release involves some movement of this granule or vesicle to the cell membrane, with which it fuses. This allows release of constituents, perhaps by ion exchange for the material to be released (Uvnäs, 1973).

Secretion usually involves activation of the cell from the external environment by a stimulus reacting with cell-surface receptors. The term "stimulus–secretion coupling" was coined to describe the events between stimulus and release (Douglas, 1968). A similarity was implied between this and the processes by which stimulus and contraction are linked ("stimulus–contraction coupling"). There is indeed great similarity. Both require ATP (energy metabolism) and Ca^{2+}. In fact, there is increasing evidence that secretion itself involves a calcium-dependent contractile process. This also appears to hold true for the release of inflammatory mediators described in this chapter. What exact role contractile, actinomyosinoid elements (microfilaments), which have now been found in most cells, play in the secretory process is at present unclear. Some hypotheses have been briefly discussed in the preceding sections.

Considerable interest has arisen in the role that cyclic nucleotides, in particular cAMP, play in cell processes. Secretion of a number of materials (e.g., hormones from the anterior pituitary, enzymes from the salivary gland, acetylcholine from the nerve endings) has been shown to be associated with increased production of cAMP. The stimulus for the release increases the activity of adenylate cyclase, and the cAMP generated, it has been postulated, acts as a "second messenger" to trigger the release process. Some questions have arisen in relation to this simple but important hypothesis. In particular, the role of Ca^{2+} and the possible antagonistic actions of cAMP and cGMP have suggested a more complex situation.

In the secretion of inflammatory mediators, cAMP (and, where studied, cGMP) also seems to play an influential although as yet undefined role. Here the situation is reversed and increased cAMP inhibits rather than enhances (or initiates) release. This difference remains unexplained. Again cGMP and cAMP may act in opposition to each other and may thus provide an important controlling influence on release.

The possible contribution to secretion of stimulus activation of serine esterases is a concept which at present is largely confined to the release of mediators. However, in view of the other similarities described, it might prove fruitful to extend the investigations to other secretory phenomena.

Many other similarities of secretion by widely different cells have been noted. Each cell also exhibits unique features. Nevertheless, it appears that a general process has become modified in different cells to produce secretion of the particular cell product. In fact, as noted above, the same general biochemical process may also have been modified to provide other cell functions such as directed movement, contraction, and phagocytosis.

Acknowledgments

I wish to fully and gratefully acknowledge the manifold contributions to this work made by Dr. Elmer L. Becker and the many hours of fruitful and exciting discussion which led to it.

9. REFERENCES

Allison, A. C., Davies, P., and DePetris, S., 1971, Role of contractile microfilaments in macrophage movement and endocytosis, *Nature New Biol.* **232:**153.

Bauer, H., Zvaifler, N. J., and Robinson, J. O., 1972, IgE immunoglobulin in the rabbit: The histopathology of the homologous passive cutaneous anaphylaxis reaction, *Lab. Invest.* 26:448.

Becker, E. L., 1972, The relationship of the chemotactic behavior of the complement-derived factors, C3a, C5a, and C̄567, and a bacterial chemotactic factor, to their ability to activate the proesterase 1 of rabbit polymorphonuclear leukocytes, *J. Exp. Med.* 135:376.

Becker, E. L., and Austen, K. F., 1966, Mechanisms of immunologic injury of rat peritoneal mast cells, *J. Exp. Med.* 124:379.

Becker, E. L., and Henson, P. M., 1973, *In vitro* studies of immunologically induced secretion of mediators from cells and related phenomena, *Advan. Immunol.* 17:93.

Becker, E. L., Showell, H. J., Henson, P. M., and Hsu, L. S., 1974, The ability of chemotactic factors to induce lysosomal enzyme release. I. The characteristics of the release, the importance of surfaces and the relation of enzyme release to chemotactic responsiveness, *J. Immunol.* 112:2047.

Benveniste, J., Henson, P. M., and Cochrane, C. G., 1973, Leukocyte dependent histamine release from rabbit platelets: The role of IgE, basophils and a platelet activating factor, *J. Exp. Med.* 136:1356.

Bodel, P., 1970, Studies on the mechanism of pyrogen production. I. Investigation of new protein synthesis in stimulated human blood leukocytes, *Yale J. Biol. Med.* 43:145.

Bokisch, V. A., Top, F. H., Russell, P. K., Dixon, F. J., and Müller-Eberhard, H. J., 1973, Pathogenic role of complement in Denque hemorrhagic shock syndrome, *New Engl. J. Med.* 289:996.

Bourne, H. R., Lehrer, R. I., Cline, M. J., and Melmon, K. L., 1971, Cyclic 3',5'-adenosine monophosphate in the human leukocyte: Synthesis, degradation and effects on neutrophil candidacidal activity, *J. Clin. Invest.* 50:920.

Bourne, H. R., Lichtenstein, L. M., and Melmon, K. L., 1972, Pharmacologic control of allergic histamine release *in vitro:* Evidence for an inhibitory role of 3',5'-adenosine monophosphate in human leukocytes, *J. Immunol.* 108:695.

Bourne, H. R., Lehrer, R. I., Lichtenstein, L. M., Weissmann, G., and Zurier, R., 1973, Effects of cholera enterotoxin on adenosine 3',5'-monophosphate and neutrophil function, *J. Clin. Invest.* 52:698.

Broder, I., 1969, Is there a common receptor for different types of antibody activating histamine histamine release in the guinea pig? in: *Cellular and Humoral Mechanisms in Anaphylaxis and Allergy* (H. Z. Movat, ed.), p. 106, Karger, Basel.

Broder, I., 1970, Comparison of histamine release by anaphylatoxin and by soluble immune complexes, *Fed. Proc.* 29:639.

Brown, D. L., and Lachmann, P. J., 1973, The behavior of complement and platelets in lethal endotoxin shock in rabbits, *Int. Arch. Allergy* 45:193.

Cox, J. P., and Karnovsky, M. L., 1973, The depression of phagocytosis by exogenous cyclic nucleotides, prostaglandins, and theophylline, *J. Cell Biol.* 59:480.

Dahlquist, R., Diamont, B., and Elwin, K., 1973, Effect of divalent cations in the interaction of adenosine 5' triphosphate (ATP) with histamine release induced by compound 48/80, *Acta Physiol. Scand.* 87:158.

David, J. R., and David, R. R., 1972, Cellular hypersensitivity and immunity, *Prog. Allergy* 16:300.

Davies, P., Rita, G. A., Krakauer, K., and Weissmann, G., 1971, Characterization of a neutral protease from lysosomes of rabbit polymorphonuclear leukocytes, *Biochem. J.* 125:559.

Davies, P., Allison, A. C., and Haswell, A. D., 1973, Selective release of lysosomal hydrolases from phagocytic cells by cytochalasin B, *Biochem. J.* 134:33.

DesPrez, D. M., and Marney, S. R., 1971, Immunological reactions involving platelets, in: *The Circulating Platelet* (S. A. Johnson, ed.), p. 415, Academic Press, New York.

Douglas, W. W., 1968, Stimulus-secretion coupling: The concept and clues from chromaffin and other cells, *Brit. J. Pharmacol.* **34**:451.

Dvorak, H. F., Dvorak, A. M., and Churchill, W. H., 1973, Immunologic rejection of diethylnitrosamine-induced hepatomas in strain 2 guinea pigs: Participation of basophilic leukocytes and macrophage aggregates, *J. Exp. Med.* **137**:751.

Estensen, R. D., Hill, H. R., Quie, P. G., Hogan, N., and Goldberg, N. D., 1973, Cyclic GMP and cell movement, *Nature (Lond.)* **254**:458.

Foreman, J. C., Mongar, J. L., and Gomperts, B. D., 1973, Calcium inophores and movement of calcium ions following the physiological stimulus to a secretory process, *Nature (Lond.)* **245**:249.

Freed, J. J., and Lebowitz, M. M., 1970, The association of a class of saltatory movements with microtubules in cultured cells, *J. Cell Biol.* **45**:334.

Gillespie, E., 1971, Colchicine binding in tissue skin, decrease by calcium and biphasic effect of adenosine 3'5'monophosphate, *J. Cell Biol.* **50**:544.

Gillespie, E., and Lichtenstein, L. M., 1972, Histamine release from human leukocytes: Studies with deuterium oxide, colchicine, and cytochalasin B, *J. Clin. Invest.* **51**:2941.

Gillespie, E., Levine, R. J., and Malawista, S. E., 1968, Histamine release from rat peritoneal mast cells: Inhibition by colchicine and potentiation by deuterium oxide, *J. Pharmacol. Exp. Ther.* **164**:158.

Goldberg, N. D., O'Dea, R. F., and Haddox, M. K., 1974, in: *Recent Advances in Cyclic Nucleotide Research* (P. Greenberg and A. G. Robison, eds.), in press, Raven Press, New York.

Goldstein, I. M., Hoffstein, S., Gallin, J., and Weissmann, G., 1973, Mechanisms of lysosomal enzyme release from human leukocytes: Microtubule assembly and membrane fusion induced by a component of complement, *Proc. Natl. Acad. Sci.* **70**:2916.

Grette, K., 1962, Studies on the mechanism of thrombin-catalyzed hemostatic reactions in blood platelets, *Acta Physiol. Scand.* **56**:Suppl. 195.

Halonen, M., Pinckard, R. N., and Meng, A. L., 1973, Characterization of IgE induced systemic anaphylaxis in the rabbit: Lack of correlation between the intravascular release of histamine and anaphylactic sensitivity, *J. Immunol.* **111**:331.

Hawkins, D., 1971, Biopolymer membrane: A model system for the study of polymorphonuclear leukocyte response to immune complexes, *J. Immunol.* **107**:344.

Hawkins, D., 1972a, Neutrophilic leukocytes in immunologic reactions: Evidence for the selective release of lysosomal constituents, *J. Immunol.* **108**:310.

Hawkins, D., 1972b, Inhibition of neutrophil lysosomal release, *Fed. Proc.* **31**:748.

Hawkins, D., and Peeters, S., 1971, The response of polymorphonuclear leukocytes to immune complexes *in vitro*, *Lab. Invest.* **24**:483.

Henney, C. S., and Bubbers, J. E., 1973, Studies on the mechanism of lymphocyte mediated cytolysis. I. The role of divalent cations in cytolysis by T lymphocytes, *J. Immunol.* **110**:63.

Henson, P. M., 1970a, Release of vasoactive amines from rabbit platelets induced by antiplatelet antibody in the presence and absence of complement, *J. Immunol.* **104**:924.

Henson, P. M., 1970b, Mechanisms of release of constituents from rabbit platelets by antigen–antibody complexes and complement. I. Lytic and nonlytic reactions, *J. Immunol.* **105**:476.

Henson, P. M., 1971a, The immunologic release of constituents from neutrophil leukocytes. I. The role of antibody and complement on nonphagocytosable surfaces or phagocytosable particles, *J. Immunol.* **107**:1535.

Henson, P. M., 1971b, The immunologic release of constituents from neutrophil leukocytes. II. Mechanisms of release during phagocytosis, and adherence to nonphagocytosable surfaces, *J. Immunol.* **107**:1547.

Henson, P. M., 1972, Pathologic mechanisms in neutrophil mediated injury, *Am. J. Pathol.* 68:593.

Henson, P. M., 1973, Mechanisms of release of granule constituents from human neutrophils phagocytosing aggregated immunoglobulin: An electron microscope study, *Arthritis Rheum.* 16:208.

Henson, P. M., and Benveniste, J., 1971, Antibody leukocyte platelet interactions, in: *Biochemistry of the Acute Allergic Reactions* (K. F. Austen and E. L. Becker, eds.), p. 111, Blackwell Scientific Publications, Oxford.

Henson, P. M., and Oades, Z. G., 1972, Enhancement of immunologically induced granule exocytosis from neutrophils by cytochalasin B, *J. Immunol.* 110:290.

Henson, P. M., and Spiegelberg, H. L., 1973, Release of serotonin from human platelets induced by aggregated immunoglobulins of different classes and subclasses, *J. Clin. Invest.* 52:1282.

Henson, P. M., Oades, Z. G., and Gould, D., 1973, Cyclic AMP and esterase activation in the release of serotonin from rabbit platelets, *Fed. Proc.* 32:1010.

Hobbs, J. B., and Cliff, W. J., 1973, A study of allograft kidney rejection occurring simultaneously in whole organ and ear chamber grafts in the rabbit, *J. Exp. Med.* 137:776.

Ignarro, L., 1973, Neutral protease release from human leukocytes regulated by neurohormones and cyclic nucleotides, *Nature New Biol.* 245:151.

Jensen, J., 1972, Anaphylatoxins, in: *Biological Activities of Complement* (D. G. Ingram, ed.), Karger, Basel.

Johnson, A. R., and Moran, N. C., 1969, Selective release of histamine from rat mast cells by compound 48/80 and antigen, *Am. J. Physiol.* 216:453.

Johnson, S. A. 1971, *The Circulating Platelet,* Academic Press, New York.

Kaliner, M., and Austen, K. F., 1973, A sequence of biochemical events in the antigen-induced release of chemical mediators from sensitized human lung tissues, *J. Exp. Med.* 138:1077.

Kaliner, M. A., Orange, R. P., Koopman, W. J., Austen, K. F., and LaRaia, P. J. 1971, Cyclic adenosine 3′,5′-monophosphate in human lung, *Biochim. Biophys. Acta* 252: 160.

Kaliner, M. A., Orange, R. P., and Austen, K. F., 1972, Immunological release of histamine and slow reacting substance of anaphylaxis from human lung, *J. Exp. Med.* 136:556.

Kay, A. B., Stechschulte, D. J., and Austen, K. F., 1971, An eosinophil leukocyte chemotactic factor of anaphylaxis, *J. Exp. Med.* 133:602.

Keller, R., 1966, in: *Tissue Mast Cells in Immune Reactions,* p. 41, American Elsevier, New York.

Kravis, T., and Henson, P. M., 1974, in preparation.

Kusner, E. J., Herzig, D. J., and Dubnick, B., 1972, *In vitro* inhibition by disodium cromoglycate (DSCG) of anaphylactic mast cell histamine release, *Fed. Proc.* 31:533.

Lagunoff, D., 1972, Contributions of electron microscopy to the study of mast cells, *J. Invest. Dermatol.* 58:296.

Lagunoff, D., 1973, Membrane fusion during mast cell secretion, *J. Cell Biol.* 57:252.

Lay, W. H., and Nussenzweig, V., 1968, Receptors for complement on leukocytes, *J. Exp. Med.* 128:991.

Levy, J. V., Cohen, J. A., and Inesi, G., 1973, Contractile effects of a calcium ionophone, *Nature (Lond.)* 242:461.

Lichtenstein, L. M., 1971, The immediate allergic response: *In vitro* separation of antigen activation, decay and histamine release, *J. Immunol.* 107:1122.

Lichtenstein, L. M., and Gillespie, E., 1973, Inhibition of histamine release by histamine controlled by H_2 receptor, *Nature (Lond.)* 244:287.

Lichtenstein, L. M., and Margolis, S., 1968, Histamine release *in vitro:* Inhibition by catecholamines and methylxanthines, *Science* 161:902.

Lucy, J. A., 1971, Biochemistry of membrane interactions, in: *Immunopathology of Inflammation* (B. K. Forscher and J. C. Houck, eds.), p. 98, Excerpta Medica, Amsterdam.

Malawista, S. E., 1971, Vinblastine: Colchicine-like effects on human blood leukocytes during phagocytosis, *Blood* 37:519.

McGuire, J., and Moellmann, G., 1972, Cytochalasin B: Effects on microfilaments and movement of melanin granules within melanocytes, *Science* 175:642.

Movat, H. Z., Uriuhara, T., Taichman, N. S., Rowsell, H. C., and Mustard, J. F., 1968, The role of PMN-leukocyte lysosomes in tissue injury inflammation and hypersensitivity. VI. The participation of the PMN-leukocyte and the blood platelet in systemic aggregate anaphylaxis, *Immunology* 14:637.

Mueller-Eckhardt, C. L., and Lüscher, E. F., 1968, Immune reactions of human blood platelets. I. A. comparative study on the effects on platelets of heterologous antiplatelet antiserum, antigen–antibody complexes, aggregated gammaglobulin and thrombin, *Thomb. Diath. Haemorrh.* 20:155.

Mustard, J. F., and Packham, M. A., 1970, Factors influencing platelet function: Adhesion, release and aggregation, *Pharm. Rev.* 22:97.

Nagayama, M., Zucker, M. B., and Beller, F. K., 1971, Effects of a variety of endotoxins on human and rabbit platelet function, *Thromb. Diath. Haemorrh.* 26:467.

Olmstead, J. B., and Borisy, G. G., 1973, Microtubules, *Ann. Rev. Biochem.* 42:507.

Orange, R. P., Austen, W. G., and Austen, K. F., 1971, Immunological release of histamine from human lung. I. Modulation by agents influencing cellular levels of cyclic 3'5'-adenosine monophosphate, *J. Exp. Med.* 134:136s.

Orr, T. S. C., Hall, D. E., and Allison, A. C., 1972, Role of contractile microfilaments in the release of histamine from mast cells, *Nature (Lond.)* 236:350.

Osler, A. G., and Siraganian, R. P., 1972. Immunologic mechanisms of platelet damage, *Prog. Allergy* 16:450.

Osler, A. G., Lichtenstein, L. M., and Levy, D. A., 1968, *In vitro* studies of human reaginic allergy, *Advan. Immunol.* 8:183.

Padawer, J., 1969, Uptake of colloidal thorium dioxide by mast cells, *J. Cell Biol.* 40:747.

Pearlman, D. S., Ward, P. A., and Becker, E. L., 1969, The requirement of serine esterase function in complement-dependent erythrocphagocytosis, *J. Exp. Med.* 130:745.

Pfueller, S. L., and Lüscher, E. F., 1972, The effects of immune complexes on blood platelets and their relationship to complement activation, *Immunochemistry* 9:1151.

Plaut, M., Lichtenstein, L. M., and Henney, C. S., 1973, Studies on the mechanism of lymphocyte-mediated cytolysis. III. The role of microfilaments and microtubules, *J. Immunol.* 110:771.

Puett, D., Wasserman, B. K., Ford, J. D., and Cunningham, L. W., 1973, Collagen-mediated platelet aggregation: Effects of collagen modification involving the protein and carbohydrate moieties, *J. Clin. Invest.* 52:2195.

Ranadive, N. S., and Cochrane, C. G., 1971, Mechanisms of histamine release from mast cells by cationic protein (band 2) from neutrophil lysosomes, *J. Immunol.* 106:506.

Rasmussen, H., 1970, Cell communication, calcium ion, and cyclic adenosine monophosphate, *Science* 170:404.

Robison, G. A., Butcher, R. W., and Sutherland, E. W., 1971, *Cyclic AMP,* Academic Press, New York.

Rubin, R. P., 1970, The role of calcium in the release of neurotransmitter substances and hormones, *Pharm. Rev.* 22:389.

Salzman, E. W., 1972, Cyclic AMP and platelet function, *New Engl. J. Med.* 286:358.

Schumaker, H. R., and Agudelo, C. A., 1971, Intravascular degranulation of neutrophils: An important factor in inflammation, *Science* 175:1139.

Scott, R. E., 1970, Effects of prostaglandins, epinephrine and Naf on human leukocyte, platelet, and liver adenyl cyclase, *Blood* 35:514.

Shibata, N., Tatsumi, N., Tanaka, K., Okamura, Y., and Senda, N., 1972, A contractile protein possessing Ca^{++} sensitivity (natural actomyosin) from leukocytes: Its extraction and some of its properties, *Biochim. Biophys. Acta* 256:565.

Shulman, N. R., Marder, V. J., Hiller, M. C., and Collier, E. M., 1964, Platelet and leukocyte isoantigens and their antibodies: Serologic, physiologic, and clinical studies, *Prog. Hematol.* 4:222.

Sneddon, J. M., 1972, Divalent cations and the platelet release reaction, *Nature (Lond.)* 236:103.

Spielvogel, A. R., 1967, An ultrastructural study of the mechanisms of platelet–endotoxin interaction, *J. Exp. Med.* 126:235.

Stechschulte, D. J., and Austen, K. F., 1973, Control mechanisms of antigen induced histamine release from rat peritoneal cells, *Int. Arch. Allergy* 45:110.

Stormorken, H., 1969, The release reaction of secretion, *Scand. J. Haematol.* 9:1.

Sullivan, A. L., Grimley, P. M., and Metzger, H., 1971, Electron microscopic localization of immunoglobulin E on the surface membrane of human basophils, *J. Exp. Med.* 134:1403.

Taylor, A., Mamelak, M., Reaven, E., and Maffly, R., 1973, Vassopressin, possible role of microtubules and microfilaments in its action, *Science* 181:347.

Tsung, P.-K., and Weissmann, G., 1973, Inhibitor of adenosine 3′,5′-monophosphate binding and protein kinase activity in leukocyte lysosomes, *Biochem. Biophys. Res. Commun.* 51:836.

Ukena, T. E., and Berlin, R. D., 1972, Effect of colchicine and vinblastine on the topographical separation of membrane functions, *J. Exp. Med.* 136:1.

Uvnäs, B., 1971, Quantitative correlation between degranulation and histamine release in mast cells, in: *Biochemistry of the Acute Allergic Reactions* (K. F. Austen and E. L. Becker, eds.), p. 175, Blackwell Scientific Publications, Oxford.

Uvnäs, B., 1973, An attempt to explain nervous transmitter release as due to nerve impulse–induced cation exchange, *Acta Physiol. Scand.* 87:168.

Valentine, M. D., Bloch, K. J., and Austen, K. F., 1967, Mechanisms of immunologic injury of rat peritoneal mast cells. III. Cytotoxic histamine release, *J. Immunol.* 99:98.

Vane, J. R., 1971, Inhibition of prostaglandin synthesis as a mechanism of action for aspirin-like drugs, *Nature New Biol.* 321:232.

Weissmann, G., and Dukor, P., 1970, The role of lysosomes in immune responses, *Advan. Immunol.* 12:283.

Weissmann, G., Dukor, P., and Zurier, R. B., 1971a, Effect of cyclic AMP on release of lysosomal enzymes from phagocytes, *Nature (Lond.)* 231:131.

Weissmann, G., Dukor, P., and Sessa, G., 1971b, Studies on lysosomes: Mechanisms of enzyme release from endocytic cells and a model for latency *in vitro*, in: *Immunopathology of Inflammation* (B. K. Forsher and J. C. Houck, eds.), p. 107, Excerpta Medica, Amsterdam.

Weismann, G., Zurier, R. B., and Hoffstein, S., 1972, Leukocytic proteases and the immunologic release of lysosomal enzymes, *Am. J. Pathol.* 68:539.

Wessels, N. K., Spooner, B. S., Ash, J. F., Bradley, M. O., Luduena, M. A., Taylor, E. L., Wrenn, J. T., and Yamada, K. M., 1971, Microfilaments in cellular and developmental processes, *Science* 171:135.

White, J. A., and Estensen, R. D., 1972, Degranulation of discoid platelets, *Am. J. Pathol.* 68:289.

White, J. G., 1971, Platelet morphology, in: *The Circulating Platelet* (S. A. Johnson, ed.), p. 46, Academic Press, New York.

Woodin, A. M., and Wieneke, A. A., 1970, Site of protein secretion and calcium accumulation in the polymorphonuclear leukocyte treated with leucocidin, in: *Calcium and Cellular Function* (A. W. Cuthbent, ed.), p. 183, Macmillan, London.

Zigmond, S., and Hirsch, J. G., 1972, Effects of cytochalasin B on polymorphonuclear leukocyte locomotion, phagocytosis and glycolysis, *Exp. Cell. Res.* 73:383.

Zucker, M. B., and Peterson, J., 1968, Inhibition of adenosine diphosphate–induced secondary aggregation and other platelet functions by acetylsalicyclic acid ingestion, *Proc. Soc. Exp. Biol. Med.* 177:547.

Zurier, R. B., Hoffstein, S., and Weissmann, G., 1973a, Cytochalasin B: Effect on lysosomal enzyme release from human leucocytes, *Proc. Natl. Acad. Sci.* 70:844.

Zurier, R. B., Hoffstein, S., and Weissmann, G., 1973b, Mechanisms of lysosomal enzyme release from human leukocytes. I. Effects of cyclic nucleotides and colchicine, *J. Cell Biol.* 58:27.

Zurier, R. B., Weissmann, G., Hoffstein, S., Kammerman, S., and Tai, H.-H., 1974, Mechanism of lysosomal enzyme release from human leukocytes. II. Effects of cyclic adenosine monophosphate and cyclic guanosine monophosphate, autonomic agonists and agents which affect microtubule function, *J. Clin. Invest.* 53:297.

LYSOSOMAL HYDROLASES AND INFLAMMATORY MATERIALS

2

Ira M. Goldstein

1. INTRODUCTION

Acute inflammatory reactions, regardless of etiology, are recognized by the presence of polymorphonuclear leukocytes at sites of tissue damage. During the past two decades, it has become appreciated that these cells are not merely innocent bystanders to the events which occur at an inflammatory site, but play an active role in the mediation of tissue injury and suppuration. Central to this role are the inflammatory substances contained within these cells, particularly those sequestered within their cytoplasmic granules, or lysosomes. The nature and mode of action of these substances are the subjects of this chapter. Particular attention will be directed toward human polymorphonuclear leukocytes and relationships between these cells and other inflammatory mediator systems in the production of human disease.

Dr. Goldstein is the recipient of an NIH Special Fellowship (1 F03 CA 55226-01) from the National Cancer Institute.

IRA M. GOLDSTEIN Department of Medicine, Division of Rheumatology, New York University School of Medicine, New York, New York.

2. POLYMORPHONUCLEAR LEUKOCYTE LYSOSOMES

2.1. Types

Originally described in rat liver (deDuve *et al.*, 1955), lysosomes are a class of subcellular organelles containing various hydrolytic enzymes, predominantly with acid pH optima, bound in latent form within a relatively impermeable membrane. The isolation and characterization of lysosomal granules from rabbit (Cohn and Hirsch, 1960*a*) and human (Hirschhorn and Weissmann, 1965) polymorphonuclear leukocytes opened an era of intensive research during which the origin, composition, and function of these organelles have been elucidated.

Bainton *et al.* (1971), for example, examined polymorphonuclear leukocytes and their precursors from normal human blood and bone marrow by histochemical staining and by electron microscopy. Based on morphological and staining characteristics, they identified two types of polymorphonuclear leukocyte granules, azurophils and specifics. Azurophil granules appeared during the promyelocyte stage of development and were observed to arise from the concave surface of the Golgi complex. These granules contained peroxidase and various other lysosomal hydrolases. Specific granules appeared during the myelocyte stage of maturation, arising from the convex face of the Golgi complex, and contained predominantly alkaline phosphatase and basic protein. The formation of azurophil granules ceased at the myelocyte stage, and this population of organelles became diluted during subsequent mitoses so that in the mature polymorph specific granules far outnumbered azurophils. These observations were analogous to those previously made in the rabbit by Bainton and Farquhar (1966, 1968*a,b*), and supported the findings of Olsson (1969), who separated human polymorphonuclear leukocyte granules on density gradients into two major subfractions: a heavy, dense granule fraction which contained acid phosphatase, β-galactosidase, and β-glucuronidase (acid hydrolases) and a heterogeneous lighter granule fraction containing all of the alkaline phosphatase. These two major granule classes, separable with regard to their content of enzymes, have recently been shown to differ in other respects as well. Nachman *et al.* (1972) observed that membranes prepared from rabbit azurophil and specific granules had similar ultrastructural appearances but differed in their content of cholesterol, phospholipid, and protein. In studies of human cells, Avila and Convit (1973*b*) found differences in physical properties between granules containing alkaline phosphatase and those containing acid hydrolases. Finally, Bainton (1973) observed that specific granules fuse with phagocytic vacuoles earlier during phagocytosis than do azurophil granules.*

* Based on these findings, and on their content of enzymes and nonenzymatic substances, specific granules are believed by some authors not to qualify as true lysosomes (Baggiolini *et al.*, 1969, 1970; Wetzel *et al.*, 1967; Bainton, 1972; Bainton and Farquhar, 1968*a*).

Other investigators have reported even greater heterogeneity than that described above among granules isolated from human and rabbit polymorphonuclear leukocytes. Welsh and Spitznagel (1971) compared the distribution of four lysosomal enzymes among subcellular fractions obtained by differential centrifugation of homogenates of human cells. They found at least three and possibly four types of lysosomes: small or low-density granules which contained acid phosphatase, large or dense granules containing peroxidase, and one or possibly two granule populations intermediate in size or density and containing lysozyme and/or β-glucuronidase. Their biochemical results were consistent with the ultrastructural observations of Watanabe *et al.* (1967) and of Daems (1968), who demonstrated three and four types of granules, respectively. For more details regarding the distribution of lysosomal enzymes among granule fractions in the rabbit, and in other species, readers are referred to Zeya and Spitznagel (1971), Folds *et al.* (1972), Farquhar *et al.* (1972), Robertson *et al.* (1972), and Avila and Convit (1973*a,b,c*).

Since the work of Cohn and Hirsch (1960*a*), numerous leukocyte lysosomal enzymes have been characterized. These enzymes, most of which are listed in a recent review by Baggiolini (1972), are capable of hydrolyzing a variety of natural and synthetic substrates. These include oligopeptides, polypeptides, simple and complex polysaccharides, phosphate esters, and lipids. A list of those enzymes which are known to be localized within human polymorphonuclear leukocyte lysosomes appears in Table I. For details and references, see Baggiolini (1972) and Avila and Convit (1973*a*).

2.2 Phagosomes, Secondary Lysosomes, pH

During phagocytosis, or particle ingestion, the granules of polymorphonuclear leukocytes fuse with invaginated portions of the plasma membrane (phagosome) and release their contents (Cohn and Hirsch, 1960*b*; Hirsch and Cohn, 1960; Hirsch, 1962; Zucker-Franklin and Hirsch, 1964). The structure that is formed, termed the "heterophagic vacuole," "phagolysosome," "phagocytic vacuole," or "secondary lysosome," serves as a digestive sac in which lysosomal enzymes are free to act on their substrates.

Considerable attention has recently been focused on the phagocytic vacuole and the changes in hydrogen ion concentration that occur within it, particularly with regard to the acidic pH optima of many of the lysosomal hydrolases. In early studies by Rous (1925), in the mouse, and by Sprick (1956), in the guinea pig, the pH of the phagocytic vacuole was found to be as low as 3.0 and 4.7, respectively. Mandell (1970) studied the changes occurring in human cells consequent to the phagocytosis of *Candida albicans* stained with indicator dyes. By 60 min, the intravacuolar pH was 6.0–6.5. The fall in pH was prevented by 20 mM sodium fluoride, 0.4 mM iodoacetate, and by refrigeration at 5°C,

Table I. Human Polymorphonuclear Leukocyte Lysosomal Enzymes

Enzyme	Hydrolytic activity (substrates)
Acid phosphatase	Orthophosphoric monoesters
α-Amylase	α-1,4-Glucan links in oligosaccharides
Laminarinase	β-1,3- or β-1,4- links adjacent to a -1,3- link in polysaccharides
Dextranase	α-1,4-Glucan links
Lysozyme	β-1,4- links between N-acetyl muramic acid and 2-acetamido-2-deoxy-D-glucose residues in a mucopolysaccharide or mucopeptide
α-Glucosidase	α-D-Glucosides
β-Glucosidase	β-D-Glucosides
β-Galactosidase	β-D-Galactosides
α-Mannosidase	α-D-Mannosides
β-Glucuronidase	β-D-Glucuronides
Aminodipeptidase	Aminoacyloligopeptides
Acid protease (Cathepsins)	Peptides
Neutral protease(s)	Peptides
Elastase	Peptides, especially at bonds adjacent to neutral amino acids
Collagenase	Native collagen
Aryl sulfhatase	Phenyl sulfates
β-N-Acetyl glucosaminidase	β-Phenyl-2-acetamido-2-deoxy-D-glucosides
Peroxidase	Hydrogen peroxide

suggesting that lactic acid production associated with the phagocytic process (Kakinuma, 1970) may have accounted for the pH change. Jensen and Bainton (1973), in similar studies employing indicator dye–stained yeast and rat peritoneal exudate leukocytes, observed a fall in pH to 6.5 within 3 min after phagocytosis, and a maximal fall to approximately 4.0 within 7–15 min. The pH changes paralleled the sequence of granule discharge (specific granules preceding azurophil granules) (Bainton, 1973), and these changes may provide a suitable milieu for the activation of lysosomal enzymes.

As discussed above, it has been suggested that the production of lactic acid is responsible for the pH change. Coffey and deDuve (1968) have suggested that the increase in vacuolar hydrogen ion concentration may result from, in part, a Donnan equilibrium associated with the presence of nondiffusable acid mucopolysaccharides within a semipermeable membrane. Recently, Cline (1973) demonstrated the presence of carbonic anhydrase in human polymorphonuclear leukocytes, and provided evidence that this enzyme may play a role in the acidification of the vacuole. Future studies will undoubtedly clarify this issue. Thus it may turn out that a proton pump keeps the vacuole acid.

3. POLYMORPHONUCLEAR LEUKOCYTES, LYSOSOMES, AND INFLAMMATION

From the foregoing discussion, it is apparent that lysosomes of polymorpho-nuclear leukocytes contain hydrolytic enzymes capable of digesting a variety of intracellular and extracellular macromolecules. These enzymes, together with other (nonenzymatic) lysosomal and nonlysosomal substances, provide polymor-phonuclear leukocytes with the necessary machinery for provoking virtually all of the features of the acute inflammatory response. Considerable experimental evidence has been accumulated to support the concept that these cells and their contents play a critical role *in vivo* in the production of inflammation and tissue injury.

Metchnikoff (1887) and later Menkin (1938) proposed that leukocytes may be involved in the liberation of substances which are capable of damaging adjacent tissues. It was not until a number of years later, however, that a crucial role for polymorphonuclear leukocytes in the production of certain experimen-tal inflammatory reactions was demonstrated. The vasculitis of the Arthus phenomenon was the first experimentally produced lesion found to be depen-dent on these cells. Specific removal of polymorphonuclear leukocytes by treatment with nitrogen mustard or heterologous antineutrophil antisera inhib-ited this reaction in several species (Stetson, 1951; Humphrey, 1955; Cochrane *et al.*, 1959; Paris, 1969; DeShazo *et al.*, 1972). Microscopically, no evidence of vascular injury could be detected in depleted animals, even though deposits of antigen, antibody, and complement could be readily demonstrated. Similarly, the necrotizing arteritis of experimental serum sickness in rabbits (Kniker and Cochrane, 1965) and the proteinuria associated with acute nephrotoxic nephritis in rats and rabbits (Cochrane *et al.*, 1965) could be prevented by depletion of polymorphonuclear leukocytes in these animals. In a recent study by Henson (1972), sheep anti-basement membrane antiserum and homologous leukocytes were injected intravenously into rabbits made neutropenic with nitrogen mus-tard. Glomerular injury resulted which varied directly with the number of polymorphonuclear leukocytes replaced by transfusion. Cells alone or antibody alone produced no glomerular damage.

Two major categories of studies implicating polymorphonuclear leukocyte lysosomes as mediators of tissue injury and inflammation have appeared. In the first category, activities of lysosomal enzymes were measured in inflammatory foci and, in the second, lysosomal lysates were tested for their capacity to produce experimental tissue damage.

Increased activities of lysosomal enzymes have been reported in human rheumatoid synovial fluid and synovial membrane, as well as in other inflamed tissues (Smith and Hamerman, 1962; Luscombe, 1963; Barland *et al.*, 1964; Lehman *et al.*, 1964; Kerby and Taylor, 1967; Coppi and Bonardi, 1968;

Barnhart *et al.*, 1968; Anderson, 1970). Morphological evidence of degranulation has been used as an indication that lysosomal enzyme release from intact leukocytes occurs *in vivo*. Henson (1972), employing ultrastructural histochemical techniques in rabbits with nephrotoxic nephritis, demonstrated alkaline phosphatase activity on the external surface of the polymorphonuclear leukocyte plasma membrane at the site of contact with the glomerular basement membrane, as well as evidence of degranulation. Schumacher and Agudelo (1972) examined small venules in human synovial membranes obtained from patients with a variety of pathological conditions (gouty arthritis, ulcerative colitis, serum sickness, rheumatoid arthritis), and observed degranulation with only occasional fragmentation of polymorphonuclear leukocytes. Vascular changes were observed to accompany degranulation: these included endothelial necrosis, gaps between endothelial cells, infiltration of the vessel wall by fibrin, and deposits of cell debris. The authors concluded that degranulation was an indication that lysosomal contents might have acted as mediators of the vascular injury.

The first direct evidence that lysosomes *per se* were capable of initiating tissue injury was provided by Thomas (1964), who found that the intradermal injection of polymorphonuclear leukocyte granules, followed by the intravenous injection of endotoxin into normal rabbits, resulted in lesions of hemorrhagic necrosis closely resembling the localized Schwartzman reaction. This treatment also enhanced skin reactivity to the reverse passive Arthus phenomenon, and made it possible to produce this reaction in neutropenic animals. Heterologous rabbit leukocyte lysosomes, when ingested by human polymorphonuclear leukocytes, produced in the host cells a series of changes culminating in cell death (Hirschhorn and Weissmann, 1967). Homologous polymorphonuclear leukocyte lysosomal lysates injected into the skin and joints of rabbits regularly produced acute inflammatory changes (Weissmann *et al.*, 1969). Repeated intra-articular injections led to hypertrophy and hyperplasia of synovial lining cells, round cell infiltration, pannus formation, and cartilage degradation. If the lystates were pretreated with heat or with ϵ-aminocaproic acid, their capacity to produce inflammation was inhibited. The lysosomal fractions were found to contain neutral protease activity capable of degrading cartilage matrix. This protease activity was similarly inhibited by ϵ-aminocaproic acid and was abolished by heating (Weissmann and Spilberg, 1968). Lysosomal lysates prepared from rabbit polymorphonuclear leukocytes have been shown to produce glomerular injury and proteinuria (ultrastructural glomerular basement membrane changes) in intact animals (Manaligod *et al.*, 1969), and both cellular detachment and digestion of rabbit corneal endothelial cells *in vitro* (Arya *et al.*, 1972).

In the sections that follow, specific lysosomal enzymes and nonenzymatic substances will be discussed with respect to their potential roles in the production of tissue injury and inflammation. Other substances, isolated from polymorphonuclear leukocytes but not necessarily confined to lysosomes, will also be discussed in this regard.

4. LYSOSOMAL ENZYMES AS INFLAMMATORY MEDIATORS

In recent years, specific lysosomal enzymes.have been isolated from polymorphonuclear leukocytes and have been found to be capable of producing tissue damage directly. These enzymes and their tissue substrates are listed in Table II, and will be discussed in the following subsections. Nonenzymatic lysosomal inflammatory substances and enzymes whose actions are mediated by way of circulating substrates will be dealt with in subsequent sections.

4.1. Acid Proteases

Historically, the acid proteases, isolated from rabbit polymorphonuclear leukocyte granules, were among the first lysosomal enzymes to be isolated and considered as important mediators of inflammation. In studies by Cohn and Hirsch (1960*a*), Lapresle and Webb (1962), Cochrane and Aiken (1966), and Wasi *et al.* (1966), these enzymes were purified and found to have properties similar to those of cathepsins D and E (tissue proteases). Cochrane and Aiken (1966) found these cathepsins capable of digesting glomerular basement membrane, at acid pH, *in vitro*. In animal experiments, however, the cathepsins failed to produce vascular injury. This was undoubtedly due to the inappropriate pH encountered by these enzymes *in vivo*.

Dingle *et al.* (1973) recently demonstrated that cathepsin D plays a major role in the intracellular digestion of certain proteins in viable cells. By employing sheep antiserum to rabbit cathepsin D, these investigators were able to inhibit

Table II. Tissue Substrates of Leukocyte Lysosomal Enzymes[a]

Substrate	Enzymes
Glomerular basement membrane	Acid protease, neutral protease, elastase
Vascular wall (Elastin)	Acid protease, neutral protease, elastase
Cartilage	Neutral protease, elastase, collagenase
Lung connective tissue	Neutral protease, elastase
Collagen	Neutral protease, collagenase

[a]For references, see text.

the intralysosomal activity of cathepsin D in intact rabbit alveolar macrophages and prevent the degradation of ingested IgG, hemoglobin, and proteoglycan.

The precise role of the acid cathepsins in the production of tissue damage and inflammation is unknown. While they probably are capable of digesting macromolecules within the confines of the phagosome, only under extreme conditions of altered tissue pH can they be expected to be active extracellularly. Whether such conditions can actually be met *in vivo* is questionable. A pH of 5.6 has been reported at an inflammatory site (Koldajew and Altschuler, 1930), but most studies have not confirmed such a dramatic change in hydrogen ion concentration. Edlow and Sheldon (1971) measured the sequential changes in pH of sterile inflammatory exudates in rabbits, and found changes which were detectable at 24 h and maximal at 72 h. The lowest mean pH was 7.049, far above the range in which acid cathepsins would be active.

4.2. Neutral Proteases

Proteolytic activity at neutral or alkaline pH had been observed in extracts of polymorphonuclear leukocytes by several investigators (Opie, 1907, 1922; Mounter and Atiyeh, 1960; Stiles and Fraenkel-Conrat, 1968; Janoff and Zeligs, 1968), but characterization of this enzyme activity lagged far behind that of the acid cathepsins. This was likely due to the fact that most investigators concentrated their efforts on cells obtained from rabbits, a species whose leukocytes possess little or no neutral protease activity (Opie, 1922; Wasi *et al.*, 1966).

Mounter and Atiyeh (1960) were perhaps the first to attempt to characterize neutral protease activity in human cells. They studied the ability of extracts prepared from human leukocytes to hydrolyze casein and denatured hemoglobin over a wide pH range and in the presence of various inhibitors. They demonstrated three sorts of proteolytic activity. Two had pH optima of 3.0 and 5.5 for the hydrolysis of casein and were thought to be derived from lymphocytes. The third enzyme had a pH optimum of 8.0 and was apparently derived from polymorphonuclear cells. This enzyme was capable of hydrolyzing acetyl tyrosine ethyl ester but not benzoyl arginine methyl ester and was inhibited by organophosphorous compounds, slightly by soybean trypsin inhibitor, and not at all by ovomucoid. These characteristics suggested that the enzyme was similar to chymotrypsin rather than to trypsin.

Further characterization of human leukocyte neutral protease activity was achieved by Janoff and Zeligs (1968). The enzyme they isolated from granule extracts digested hemoglobin and N-benzyloxycarbamyl-L-alanine-p-nitrophenyl ester (NBA ester) at neutral pH. These activities were not affected by specific inhibitors of trypsin, chymotrypsin, and cathepsins B and C (neutral proteases). Furthermore, synthetic substrates for trypsin and chymotrypsin were not hydrolyzed by the leukocyte enzyme. When granule extracts containing this neutral protease activity were injected into normal rabbits, lesions similar to that of an Arthus reaction resulted. Protease inhibitors obtained from soybean or salivary gland prevented these lesions when administered with the granule extracts. *In vitro* studies demonstrated the ability of these extracts to lyse rabbit glomerular basement membrane at neutral pH.

Despite earlier reports to the contrary (Cohn and Hirsch, 1960a; Cochrane and Aiken, 1966), a neutral protease from lysosomes of rabbit polymorphonuclear leukocytes has been isolated and characterized (Davies *et al.*, 1971, 1972). This enzyme, which is optimally active between pH 7.0 and 7.5, hydrolyzes calf thymus histone but not hemoglobin or synthetic substrates for trypsin and chymotrypsin. The enzyme is associated with azurophil granules and is readily inhibited by a cytoplasmic factor. The effect of the cytosol inhibitor was reversed by increasing the ionic strength of the medium, and by polyanions such as heparin and dextran sulfate. Human serum and fetal calf serum completely inhibited this neutral protease activity.

It is apparent from the foregoing discussion that lysosomal neutral proteases may play a significant role in the mediation of tissue damage and inflammation. Recent studies regarding the action of these enzymes on two important substrates, elastin and collagen, will be discussed in the following sections.

4.3. Human Leukocyte Elastase-like Esterase

Janoff and Sherer (1968), employing orcein-dyed elastin as substrate, demonstrated elastinolytic activity in a neutral protease fraction obtained from human polymorphonuclear leukocyte lysosomes. The enzyme had optimal activity at pH 8.5 but retained approximately half of this activity in the pH range of 6.0–7.0. Elastinolytic activity was inhibited somewhat by dilute human serum as well as by soybean trypsin inhibitor and salivary gland kallikrein inhibitor, but not by high salt concentration or EDTA. These and other properties of the enzyme, which the authors termed "leukocyte-elastase," differed considerably from those of pancreatic elastases. Furthermore, the elastinolytic activity could be separated from collagenase activity (see below) by ion exchange chromatography. Treatment of frozen sections of human kidney and strips of renal artery with crude enzyme fractions produced alterations in staining properties of the elastica of arterial vessels and partial fragmentation of the internal elastic lamina, resembling the changes associated with acute arteritis. Using a more purified enzyme, Janoff (1970) was able to produce similar changes in canine aortas *in vivo*. This preparation also solubilized human renal basement membrane, and when injected into rabbit skin produced vascular injury and local hemorrhage. Similar enzyme preparations have been shown to release protein from rabbit articular cartilage (Janoff and Blondin, 1970) and from insoluble connective tissue fractions prepared from human lung (Janoff *et al.,* 1972). A peptide chloromethyl ketone inhibitor of elastase failed to inhibit the activity of granule extracts on cartilage and renal basement membrane, whereas activity against arterial wall and connective tissue fractions from human lung was completely inhibited (Janoff, 1972*a*). These results suggest that other lysosomal neutral proteases may play a dominant role in degrading cartilage and renal basement membrane, whereas arterial walls and lung tissue are susceptible to hydrolysis by the elastase-like enzyme.

Two potent natural inhibitors of this elastinolytic enzyme have been characterized. One is a factor present in human leukocyte cytosol fractions (analogous to the rabbit neutral protease inhibitor) and the other is serum α_1-antitrypsin. The cytosol inhibitor (Janoff and Blondin, 1971) does not affect pancreatic elastase and is not antigenically related to α_1-antitrypsin or α_2-macroglobulin. It is thermolabile and inactivated by pronase. α_1-Antitrypsin inhibits human leukocyte neutral proteolytic activity in general (Kueppers and Bearn, 1966) and is a potent inhibitor of the elastase-like enzyme (Ohlsson, 1971; Janoff, 1972*b*; Lieberman and Kaneshiro, 1972). The elastase–α_1-antitrypsin complex migrates as a β-globulin, whereas the neutral protease–α_1-antitrypsin complex migrates as an α_3-globulin on agarose gel electrophoresis (Ohlsson, 1971), providing, perhaps, additional evidence that the elastase-like enzyme is distinctive. α_2-Macroglobulin (plasmin inhibitor) is a less effective elastase inhibitor but may be important in α_1-antitrypsin deficiency states (Janoff, 1972*b*).

4.4. Human Leukocyte Collagenase

Collagenases are enzymes which cleave native collagen molecules in a characteristic fashion to yield two specific products which have been termed "TC^A" and "TC^B." The TC^A fragment is the N-terminal three-quarter-length product, and the TC^B fragment is the C-terminal one-quarter-length product (Kang *et al.,* 1966). A specific collagenase, active at neutral and alkaline pH, has been found in granule fractions from human polymorphonuclear leukocytes (Lazarus *et al.,* 1968*a*). This leukocyte collagenase was inhibited by EDTA, cysteine, and reduced glutathione, but not by human serum, distinguishing it from previously described tissue collagenases and from other neutral proteases (Lazarus *et al.,* 1968*b*) of leukocytes. Incubation of collagen with crude granule extracts at neutral pH results in cleavage of the collagen molecules into two specific products as well as to extensive lysis of fibrils. Purification of collagenase activity results in the enzyme's loss of ability to solubilize collagen fibrils, although cleavage of the collagen molecule into TC^A and TC^B fragments still takes place. The degradative activity, lost during purification, was identified as due to a nonspecific protease system. The protease can be inhibited by serum, a cytosol factor, soybean trypsin inhibitor, and diisopropyl fluorophosphate. In addition to degrading TC^A and TC^B fragments, this protease system may independently hydrolyze collagen to some extent. For maximal collagen degradation, however, both the specific collagenase and the protease system are required (Lazarus *et al.*, 1972).

4.5. Neutral Proteases and Human Disease

The long list of potential substrates for neutral protases of leukocytes makes these enzymes excellent candidates for important mediators of tissue injury and inflammation. In some patients with rheumatoid arthritis, for example, leukocyte elastase (Janoff and Blondin, 1970) and collagenase (Harris *et al.*, 1969) have been isolated from synovial fluid. It is easy to picture how these neutral proteases may play a role in producing vascular and glomerular damage in such disorders as polyarteritis nodosa, systemic lupus erythematosus, glomerulonephritis, serum sickness, etc. However, the disease process that has been studied most extensively in terms of the pathogenetic role played by leukocyte proteases is emphysema. Elastin is the major connective tissue determinant of lung structure and elastic behavior (Johanson and Pierce, 1972). Destruction of elastin and other connective tissue elements of lung, by papain, for example, produces lesions similar to those seen in naturally occurring emphysema (Pushpakom *et al.*, 1970). That leukocyte enzymes are capable of producing similar pathological changes has been determined by several investigators. Marco *et al.* (1971) administered aerosolized homogenates of dog leukocytes intratracheally and produced dilation of terminal airways with destruction and loss of alveoli. Animals treated with homogenates that were heated to destroy protease activity did not develop lesions. Mass *et al.* (1972) found that homogenates of polymorphonuclear leukocytes from dogs and humans, as opposed to homogenates from rabbit polymorphonuclear and dog mononuclear leukocytes, were capable of producing emphysema-like lesions. The ability of the cell homogenates to induce experimental emphysema correlated with the presence of neutral and alkaline protease activity *in vitro*. Similarly, leukocyte proteases from purulent sputum were found capable of digesting human lung tissue *in vitro* (Lieberman and Gawad, 1971). Thus evidence has accumulated to support the hypothesis that leukocyte proteases play a role in the pathogenesis of pulmonary emphysema. Further support for this hypothesis has been based on the observation that individuals genetically deficient in α_1-antitrypsin are particularly prone to develop emphysema (Eriksson, 1964). Though α_1-antitrypsin has little effect on the weak elastase-like proteolytic activity found in human alveolar macrophage granules (Janoff *et al.*, 1971) or on leukocyte collagenase activity (Lazarus *et al.*,

1972), it is a potent inhibitor of other neutral proteases found in human polymorphonuclear leukocytes and in purulent sputum (Ohlsson, 1971; Lieberman and Gawad, 1971; Janoff, 1972*b*; Lieberman and Kaneshiro, 1972). Thus in the presence of deficient levels of α_1-antitrypsin, leukocyte proteases are free to attack the lung parenchyma and produce the destructive lesions associated with emphysema.

The concept that pulmonary disease may result from an imbalance between protease and antiprotease activities has recently gained support from studies performed by Galdston *et al.* (1973). These investigators measured levels of leukocyte lysosomal elastase-like esterase activity in family members of patients with deficiencies of serum α_1-antitrypsin, and related them to levels of nonspecific neutral protease (denatured hemoglobin as substrate) and β-glucuronidase activities and to the patients' clinical status. There was a good correlation between esterase and neutral protease activity, but neither was related to β-glucuronidase activity. Two levels of activity of these enzymes were detected, one similar to that measured in a control group and the other one-half this level. An unfavorable clinical course was observed in those individuals with normal levels of enzyme activity associated with intermediate-low or low trypsin inhibitory capacity. These findings suggest that the degree of leukocyte lysosomal protease–antiprotease imbalance in patients with α_1-antitrypsin deficiency might determine the clinical expression of pulmonary disease.

A summary of the possible roles played by leukocyte neutral proteases in human disease is presented in Fig. 1.

5. NONENZYMATIC INFLAMMATORY MEDIATORS

Among the inflammatory mediators contained within polymorphonuclear leukocytes are a group of substances without known enzymatic activity. These include lysosomal cationic proteins and histamine. Two other substances, to be discussed below, are not capable of directly producing tissue injury but nevertheless mediate the systemic effects which often accompany a localized inflammatory response.

5.1. Cationic Proteins

A heterogeneous group of basic (cationic) proteins, devoid of enzymatic activity, have been isolated from rabbit polymorphonuclear leukocyte lysosomes. These proteins have diverse biological activities (Table III), and are capable of either directly or indirectly producing tissue damage and inflamma-

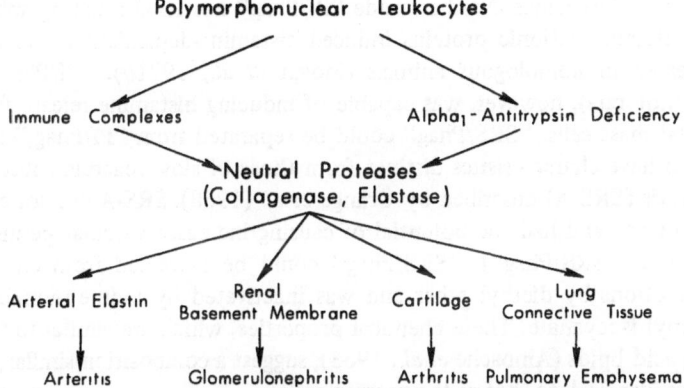

Fig. 1. Neutral proteases and human disease.

tion. They caused adhesion and extravascular emigration of leukocytes, and petechial hemorrhages in the microcirculation of the rat and rabbit mesentery (Janoff and Zweifach, 1964) and an acute inflammatory response in rabbit skin (Golub and Spitznagel, 1966). In subsequent studies, specific cationic protein fractions were found to be capable of inducing histamine release from mast cells (Seegers and Janoff, 1966; Scherer and Janoff, 1968; Ranadive and Cochrane, 1968) and of producing marked (histamine-independent) capillary permeability changes directly (Ranadive and Cochrane, 1968). Recently, Movat *et al.* (1971a) demonstrated that peritoneal polymorphonuclear leukocytes of rabbits, guinea pigs, and rats incubated *in vitro* with antigen–antibody precipitates released a substance, termed "Pf/Phag," which enhanced vascular permeability and in high concentrations caused hemorrhage when injected intradermally into the same species. These effects were not inhibited by antihistamines. Another substance, "SRS/Phag," was released under similar conditions and induced a slow contraction of guinea pig ileum and rat uterus. Both substances were shown to be

Table III. Biological Activities of
Lysosomal Cationic Proteins

Enhancement of vascular permeability
Histamine release from mast cells
Chemotactic
Anticoagulant
Coagulant
Antiheparin
Pyrogenic
Antibacterial

derived from lysosomes. Neither crude "Pf/Phag" nor its chromatographic fractions containing cationic proteins induced histamine-dependent vascular injury when tested in homologous animals (Movat *et al.*, 1971*b*). "Pf/Phag" from rabbits (not rats), however, was capable of inducing histamine release from rat peritoneal mast cells. "SRS/Phag" could be separated from "Pf/Phag," and was shown to have characteristics distinct from those of slow reacting substance of anaphylaxis (SRS-A) described by Orange *et al.* (1968). SRS-A did not contract the rat uterus and had the potential of causing increased vascular permeability (opposed to "SRS/Phag"). "SRS/Phag" could be extracted from crude lysosomal fractions by diethyl ether and was inactivated by iodine monobromide and phenyl isocyanate. These chemical properties, which are similar to those of hydroxyacid lipids (Ambache *et al.*, 1963), suggest a composition similar, but by no means identical, to that of the prostaglandins.

Lysosomal cationic protein fractions derived from rabbit polymorphonuclear leukocytes have other biological activities. These include anticoagulant (Saba *et al.*, 1967), procoagulant (Hawiger *et al.*, 1969*a*), and antiheparin (Poplawski *et al.*, 1969) activities. In addition, they may be pyrogenic (Herion *et al.*, 1966), chemotactic (Ward, 1968), and bactericidal (Zeya and Spitznagel, 1966, 1968). Recently, Hawiger *et al.* (1972) have shown that cationic proteins are capable of complexing with artificial membranes (liposomes), preventing them from activating lysosomal enzymes in intact leukocyte granules (Hawiger *et al.*, 1969*b*). It has been suggested that these proteins may serve an *in vivo* function by controlling the activity of lysosomal enzymes. Other recent developments in the study of these proteins include the finding that, at high concentrations, they inhibit respiration in rat liver mitochondria, possibly (as suggested) due to their effects on mitochondrial membrane integrity and their ability to interfere with electron transport by inhibiting cytochrome oxidase (Penniall and Zeya, 1971; Penniall *et al.*, 1972).

The role of lysosomal cationic proteins in producing human disease is unknown. These proteins can be isolated from human polymorphonuclear leukocytes but, in general, do not share the properties of similar proteins isolated from other species, particularly the rabbit. For example, attempts to demonstrate pyrogenic (Herion *et al.*, 1966) or vascular permeability enhancing activities (Scherer and Janoff, 1968) in fractions of human lysosomal cationic proteins have failed. The antibacterial activity of these proteins will be discussed in a subsequent section.

5.2. Histamine

Among the nonenzymatic inflammatory mediators contained within leukocytes is the potent vasoactive agent, histamine. Since a more complete discussion of this substance appears in Chapter 5, the remarks in this section will be limited to a brief description of recent work regarding the histamine content of leukocytes and certain factors relating to its release from these cells.

Graham *et al.* (1955) are credited with providing the first evidence that human polymorphonuclear leukocytes contain significant amounts of histamine. This view, however, was not supported by subsequent investigators (Simpson and Archer, 1967; Pruzansky and Patterson, 1970), who have argued that histamine is confined almost exclusively to basophils and eosinophils in mixed leukocyte suspensions. Despite this controversy regarding the relative contribution made by polymorphonuclear leukocytes to total leukocyte histamine, evidence remains that these cells do contain this inflammatory mediator.

Crowder *et al.* (1969) observed that phagocytosis of opsonized staphylococci by normal human polymorphonuclear leukocytes was associated with release into the extracellular medium of histamine and the lysosomal enzymes, lysozyme and cathepsins. These events were not associated with changes in cell viability. Kelly *et al.* (1971a) found that when dog polymorphonuclear leukocyte lysates were administered intravenously to normal dogs, increased plasma histamine levels resulted. These same authors (Kelly *et al.*, 1971b) found that lysates of human polymorphonuclear leukocytes, platelets, and lymphocytes released histamine from intact human leukocytes *in vitro*. The histamine-releasing activity was equally distributed between lysosomal and supernatant fractions of these lysates, and could be separated from lysosomal cationic proteins.

Human leukocyte histamine has been observed to be granule associated and to have a similar, although not identical, subcellular distribution as lysosomal β-glucuronidase (Pruzansky and Patterson, 1967). Evidence that these two substances are probably not contained within the same class of granules was obtained by May *et al.* (1970), who demonstrated that the antigen-induced release of histamine from sensitive human leukocytes was not accompanied by release of β-glucuronidase. These investigators also found that the extrusion of β-glucuronidase after phagocytosis of zymosan particles occurred without simultaneous release of histamine.

5.3. Leukocyte Pyrogen

Although not necessarily an inflammatory mediator, leukocyte pyrogen plays an important role in determining the systemic response to tissue injury and bacterial invasion. Beeson (1948) was the first to observe that rabbit leukocytes were capable of releasing a pyrogenic substance when appropriately stimulated. In later work, Bennett and Beeson (1953) demonstrated pyrogen in the supernatant fraction of disrupted rabbit polymorphonuclear leukocytes. Detailed studies of human leukocyte pyrogen (Cranston *et al.*, 1956) were made possible when Bodel and Atkins (1966) determined that a substance from human polymorphonuclear leukocytes was capable of producing fever in rabbits. This observation established that the activity of leukocyte pyrogen was not species specific and provided a convenient system for assaying human material.

Human (and rabbit) peripheral blood polymorphonuclear leukocytes, in contrast to rabbit exudate leukocytes, release little or no pyrogen when incubated in buffer solutions unless previously activated by exposure to bacterial endotoxin or by being provided with a phagocytic stimulus (e.g., heat-killed staphylococci) (Bodel, 1970; Moore et al., 1970; Root et al., 1970). Following either stimulus there is a variable latent period, after which pyrogen release occurs. Inhibition of protein or RNA synthesis during this period prevents pyrogen release. Moore et al. (1973) incubated stimulated rabbit leukocytes in the presence of radiolabeled amino acids and were able to demonstrate, during the activation stage, incorporation of radioactivity into new protein which was pyrogen. The activation process in human leukocytes is also thought to involve the synthesis of new cellular protein, but experiments have thus far failed to prove this conclusively (Bodel, 1970). Pyrogen released from rabbit polymorphonuclear leukocytes is probably not derived from their granules (Hahn et al., 1970). Virtually all of the preformed pyrogen that could be extracted from sucrose-lysed cells was found in the cytoplasmic fraction. These results were contrary to those of Herion et al. (1966), who were able to demonstrate pyrogenicity in a lysosomal cationic protein fraction.

5.4. Leukocytic Endogenous Mediator

Extracts of rat polymorphonuclear leukocytes, prepared according to the methods commonly used to prepare endogenous pyrogen, produced dose-dependent reductions in both serum zinc and iron concentrations in the intact rat

Table IV. Circulating Substrates of Leukocyte Lysosomal Enzymes[a]

Substrate	Enzyme	Biological activity
C5	Neutral protease	Chemotaxis (?anaphylatoxin)
C3	Neutral protease	Chemotaxis (?)
Cīs	?	Complement inactivation
Fibrin	Neutral protease (?) Acid protease	Fibrinolysis
Plasminogen	Plasminogen activator	Fibrinolysis
Leukokininogen	Acid protease	Leukokinins
Kinins	Kininase (acid protease)	Kinin inactivation

[a]For references, see text.

without evoking a febrile response (Kampschmidt and Upchurch, 1969, 1970; Pekarek and Beisel, 1971). The active substance, termed "leukocytic endogenous mediator," was found to be a heat-labile, nondialyzable, low molecular weight protein, similar in many respects to endogenous pyrogen (Pekarek and Beisel, 1971), but differing in species specificity and susceptibility to proteolytic enzymes (Pekarek *et al.*, 1972). This hormone-like factor, which has been demonstrated in the serum of infected humans and experimental animals, not only affects trace metal metabolism but also depresses serum amino acid levels by causing a net flux of amino acids into liver tissue, and stimulates hepatic RNA and protein synthesis (Wannemacher *et al.*, 1972*a,b*; Pekarek *et al.*, 1973).

6. LEUKOCYTE-DERIVED SUBSTANCES AND INFLAMMATORY MEDIATOR SYSTEMS

The preceding sections of this chapter were primarily concerned with substances contained within leukocytes that are capable of directly producing tissue damage. This section is devoted to a discussion of cell-derived substances (mostly enzymes) that do not affect tissues directly but interact with other inflammatory mediator systems through their actions on circulating substrates (Table IV). It should become clear that, through such interactions, mechanisms exist for both the propagation and the amplification of the inflammatory response. Some of the mediator systems mentioned below will be described in greater detail in subsequent chapters, i.e., the complement system and the kinins.

6.1. Complement and Mediators of Chemotaxis

The extravascular migration and accumulation of polymorphonuclear leukocytes at sites of tissue injury are hallmarks of the inflammatory response. Considerable experimental evidence has been gathered in support of the view that chemotaxis plays a significant role in leukocyte accumulation at inflammatory sites. Chemotaxis has been defined as a reaction by which the direction of cellular locomotion is determined by chemical substances in the environment (McCutcheon, 1946). That such substances may be derived from leukocytes directly or generated extracellularly by leukocyte enzymes is the subject of the following discussion.

Hurley (1964) provided perhaps the earliest evidence that one or more substances within leukocytes either possessed chemotactic activity or were capable of generating such activity. He found that saline extracts of polymorphonuclear leukocytes stimulated leukocyte migration *in vivo* and *in vitro*.

Increased stimulatory activity was obtained if the cells were incubated in fresh serum. Cell-derived, serum-independent chemotactic activity was subsequently described by several authors (Cornely, 1966; Ward, 1968; Borel *et al.*, 1969). In each instance, activity was localized in leukocyte lysosomal fractions. The chemotactic activity derived from these lysosomal lysates was generally weak except for the material isolated from polymorphonuclear leukocytes by Ward (1968), which was markedly chemotactic for mononuclear cells. Phelps (1969) was able to demonstrate modest amounts of serum-independent chemotactic activity in supernatants of suspensions of polymorphonuclear leukocytes and monosodium urate crystals, and determined that phagocytosis was a prerequisite for the appearance of this activity.

Zigmond and Hirsch (1973) described a heat-stable, nondialyzable serum-independent chemotactic factor released into the suspending medium by human polymorphonuclear leukocytes exposed to heat-aggregated γ-globulin fixed to glass.

The finding that enhanced chemotactic activity was obtained when whole cell or lysosomal lysates were incubated in fresh serum (Hurley, 1964; Borel *et al.*, 1969) suggested the presence of an inactive substrate in serum which could be acted on by an enzyme or enzymes contained within lysosomes to yield chemotactic activity. One such substrate has been identified as the fifth component of complement. Ward and Hill (1970) identified a lysosomal enzyme obtained from rabbit polymorphonuclear leukocytes that was capable of cleaving human C5 (not human C3) into chemotactically active fragments of variable molecular weights. The enzyme acted at neutral pH and was inhibited by esters bearing basic amino acids, ε-aminocaproic acid, soybean trypsin inhibitor, and EDTA. It was clearly not identical with a tissue protease which could produce C3-derived leukotactic factors (Hill and Ward, 1969, 1971). A similar enzyme, acting at neutral pH, was described in human polymorphonuclear leukocyte lysosomes (Taubman *et al.*, 1970). This enzyme, when incubated with either purified C5 or fresh human serum, generated chemotactic activity similar to that generated by immunological activation of the complement system. This lysosomal enzyme was also capable of cleaving C3 into large and small fragments. A proteinase with an acid pH optimum has recently been isolated from macrophages and is also capable of cleaving C5 into a number of fragments chemotactic for polymorphonuclear leukocytes and mononuclear cells (Snyderman *et al.*, 1972). Though precise identification of the leukotactic fragments generated by these enzymes is lacking, it is likely that some are identical to human C5a. This complement component is known to be a potent chemotactic factor (Ward and Newman, 1969) and possesses anaphylatoxin activity as well (Cochrane and Muller-Eberhard, 1968). C5a has recently been shown to be capable of mediating lysosomal enzyme release from human polymorphonuclear leukocytes (Goldstein *et al.*, 1973), thereby providing a mechanism for its own generation as well as for the propagation and amplification of the inflammatory response.

Additional mechanisms whereby leukocytes may participate in the generation of chemotactic activity are related to their capacity to mediate fibrinolysis (see below) and collagenolysis. Fibrin split products (Stecher and Sorkin, 1972), degradation products of collagen (Houck and Chang, 1971), and products of the action of plasmin on C3 (Ward, 1967) are all chemotactic.

Leukocyte-derived substances may affect cell locomotion in other ways. A neutrophil-immobilizing factor described by Goetzl and Austen (1972) irreversibly inhibits the response of human polymorphonuclear leukocytes to diverse chemotactic stimuli without impairing their viability. Although the subcellular localization of this low molecular weight (approximately 5000) factor is unknown, it appears to exist in a preformed state in human polymorphonuclear leukocytes and mononuclear cells. It is released from these cells in an acid medium, after exposure to bacterial endotoxin and then incubation in a hypokalemic medium, and during phagocytosis of particles. Another, perhaps related, low molecular weight human leukocyte–derived factor inhibits the random migration of guinea pig peritoneal macrophages (Statsny and Ziff, 1970). Finally, inhibition of complement-derived chemotactic factor generation may be mediated by one or more enzymes present in human polymorphonuclear leukocyte lysosomes which are capable of inactivating the esteratic function of C1s̄, the active moiety of the first component of complement (Taubman and Lepow, 1971).

6.2. Coagulation and Fibrinolytic Systems

The participation of components of the blood coagulation and fibrinolytic systems in the inflammatory response has been recently reviewed by McKay (1972), and the relationships between these systems and the complement and kinin systems will be discussed in subsequent chapters. The following discussion will be limited to those aspects of coagulation and fibrinolysis mediated in part, or solely, by leukocytes.

The deposition of fibrin either intravascularly or in tissue spaces plays a major role in some inflammatory reactions. In addition to directly producing tissue injury by ischemia, fibrin limits the spread of invading microorganisms and provides a framework for migrating cells and for reparative connective tissue.

6.2.1. Coagulation

Jones (1851) is credited with first suggesting that leukocytes might be involved in blood coagulation at sites of vascular injury. It was not until recently, however, that mechanisms for such involvement became apparent. Rapaport and Hjort (1967) observed that intact rabbit polymorphonuclear leukocytes possessed coagulant activity resembling that of tissue thromboplastin.

In subsequent studies, similar coagulant activity was found in human and canine leukocytes (Erdogan, 1968; Lerner et al., 1971; Kociba et al., 1972; Saba et al., 1973).

The activity is generally not present in freshly collected human leukocytes, but appears during in vitro incubation in plasma or serum. Exposure of leukocytes to bacterial endotoxin results in enhancement of both its activity and its rate of appearance (Lerner et al., 1971), effects which are inhibited by actinomycin D, puromycin, and cycloheximide (Niemetz, 1972a). Endotoxin may also play a role in vivo in enhancing leukocyte coagulant activity. When rabbit peritoneal leukocytes were obtained from animals which had received two spaced doses of endotoxin, significant thromboplastin-like activity was released from these cells after only 15 min of incubation in buffer (Niemetz, 1972b). When these leukocytes were infused into aortas of normal rabbits, extensive generalized intravascular coagulation occurred and typical lesions of the generalized Shwartzman reaction were observed (Niemetz and Fani, 1971). Lysates of rabbit leukocytes which had been incubated in vitro for 24 h produced similar lesions when infused intra-aortically into normal rabbits (Kociba and Griesemer, 1972). Though the precise subcellular localization of leukocyte coagulant activity is unknown, there is evidence to suggest an association with lysosomes. Niemetz (1972b) assayed fractions of rabbit peritoneal leukocytes obtained by centrifugation of homogenates and found thromboplastin-like activity in the $14,500g$ sediment, suggesting that the bulk of activity was perhaps granule associated. Kociba et al. (1972) and Saba et al. (1973), in their studies of human leukocytes, similarly found coagulant activity in granule fractions. Further evidence implicating leukocyte granules as the source of coagulant activity was provided by Horn and Collins (1968). In their studies, isolated granules infused into normal rabbits with a single dose of endotoxin resulted in intravascular coagulation. Intravenous administration produced thromboses in the pulmonary vasculature, whereas intra-aortic administration resulted in renal cortical necrosis and lesions typical of the generalized Shwartzman reaction. That the coagulant activity may be associated with lysosomal membranes is evidenced by its resistance to solubilization in granule fractions (Kociba et al., 1972) and by the observation that phospholipids extracted from human leukocytes possess thromboplastic activity (Erdogan, 1968).

Though unrelated to the coagulant activity discussed above, another lysosomal constituent has been found which may be important in producing intravascular fibrin deposition. Hawiger et al. (1969a) isolated a lysosomal cationic protein fraction from rabbit polymorphonuclear leukocytes that had antiheparin activity and was capable of precipitating soluble fibrin monomer complexes nonenzymatically. Antiheparin activity has also been isolated from rabbit leukocytes by Saba et al. (1968) and from human leukocytes by Poplawski et al. (1969).

Lysosomal cationic proteins isolated from human and rabbit polymorphonuclear leukocytes have been found to possess anticoagulant activity (Martin and Roka, 1951; Saba *et al.*, 1967). This heterogeneous group of proteins did not inhibit clotting factors directly, but rather they were shown to interfere with the formation of intrinsic thromboplastin.

6.2.2. Fibrinolysis

Rulot (1904) reported that fibrin dissolution in saline was greatly accelerated if leukocytes were present in the fibrin network. He was the first to suggest that fibrinolysis may result from the release of leukocyte-bound proteolytic enzymes. Just a few years after this suggestion, Opie (1907) described a leukoprotease derived from polymorphonuclear leukocytes which was capable of digesting coagulated blood, fibrin, gelatin, and casein. Numerous reports subsequently appeared describing the biochemical characteristics of this protease (Gans, 1963; Astrup *et al.*, 1967; Barnhart *et al.*, 1968; Prokopowicz, 1968; Prokopowicz and Stormorken, 1968). In recent years, several investigators have demonstrated that leukocytes also contain plasminogen, as well as plasminogen activator (Gans, 1963; Lack and Ali, 1964; Saba *et al.*, 1969; Matsuoka *et al.*, 1969; Goldstein *et al.*, 1971).

Electron and fluorescent microscopic studies of leukocytes migrating into areas of experimentally induced inflammation have revealed involvement of lysosomal granules in the digestion of fibrin deposited at the inflammatory site (Riddle and Barnhart, 1964; Barnhart, 1965). Evidence for the localization of plasminogen activator activity within lysosomes came from the work of Saba *et al.* (1969), who identified this enzyme in a lysosomal cationic protein fraction isolated from rabbit and human polymorphonuclear leukocytes. Furthermore, in studies based on the enhancing effect of bacterial endotoxins on the release of hydrolytic enzymes from lysosome preparations, Lack (1963) effected the release of plasminogen activator from isolated rabbit leukocyte lysosomes. Endotoxin has also been shown to stimulate the release of this enzyme from intact, viable human polymorphonuclear leukocytes, paralleling the release of lysosomal β-glucuronidase (Goldstein *et al.*, 1971; Wunschmann-Henderson *et al.*, 1972).

It is difficult to assess the relative contribution made by leukocytes toward the dissolution of fibrin *in vivo*, although one can speculate that it may be substantial in an inflammatory exudate. Gans (1963) and Lack (1963) have suggested that leukocytes may account for a considerable fraction of plasma fibrinolytic activity.

6.3. Leukokinins

Kinins, as mediators of inflammation, will be discussed in greater detail in Chapter 3. The role of leukocytes in the generation of kinin activity, however, deserves mention here.

Leukokinins are pharmacologically active peptides which are produced by leukocyte enzymes acting on plasma substrates at acidic pH. The peptides are very active as hypotensive agents by relaxing arteriolar smooth muscle, and as agents which increase vascular permeability (Freer *et al.*, 1972), hence their role as inflammatory mediators. That leukocytes of the granulocytic series contained kinin-forming enzymes was determined by Greenbaum and Kim (1967) and by Melmon and Cline (1967). The latter investigators found that the addition of human polymorphonuclear leukocytes to plasma or serum resulted in a two- to threefold increase in kinin concentration within 5 min. Kinin generation was inhibited by cortisol and appeared to require an intact glycolytic pathway as well as protein and RNA synthesis. Subsequently, Melmon and Cline (1968) reported that human polymorphonuclear leukocytes, as well as neoplastic cells and eosinophils, possessed both kinin-generating and kininase activities. They provided evidence that at acid pH kinin-generating activity was associated with granule fractions obtained from these cells, and suggested possible roles for Hageman factor and kallikrein in the system, making it analogous to the plasma kinin-generating system. The leukocyte kinin-generating system, however, has been subsequently shown to be quite different from the well-known bradykinin-generating system of plasma.

The leukocyte enzymes (leukokininogenases) capable of generating kinin activity are acid proteases, with a pH optimum of 4.0, whereas kallikrein acts at neutral pH (Greenbaum and Kim, 1967). Leukokininogenases are not inhibited by Trasylol, are not or only partially inhibited by soybean trypsin inhibitor, and are probably present within the cell in an active form. Leukokininogenase activity is membrane bound and is found in lysosomal and nonlysosomal fractions, whereas leukocyte kininase is not granule associated (Greenbaum, 1972). Leukokininogen in human plasma is distinct from bradykininogen, the substrate for kallikrein, and is normally present as such only in small amounts. Increased amounts of leukokininogen as available substrate, however, can be generated from an unknown precursor (unavailable substrate) by the activation of a plasma protease (?kallikrein-like enzyme) (Greenbaum *et al.*, 1972; Greenbaum, 1972). Greenbaum *et al.* (1969) introduced the term "PMN-kinin" to describe the polypeptide differing from bradykinin or its analogues which was generated from human plasma kininogen by the leukokininogenase(s) of human polymorphonuclear leukocytes. Two pharmacologically active peptides have now been isolated from incubation mixtures of human kininogen and enzyme fractions obtained from rabbit macrophages and polymorphonuclear leukocytes. The peptides have been partially sequenced, and although they have properties similar to those of bradykinin, they do not contain bradykinin as part of their molecules. Leukokinin-M (macrophage enzyme mediated) contains 25 amino acids and has a molecular weight of 2826.5 daltons. Leukokinin-PMN (polymorphonuclear leukocyte enzyme mediated) has 21 amino acids (mol wt 2145) (Chang *et al.*, 1972).

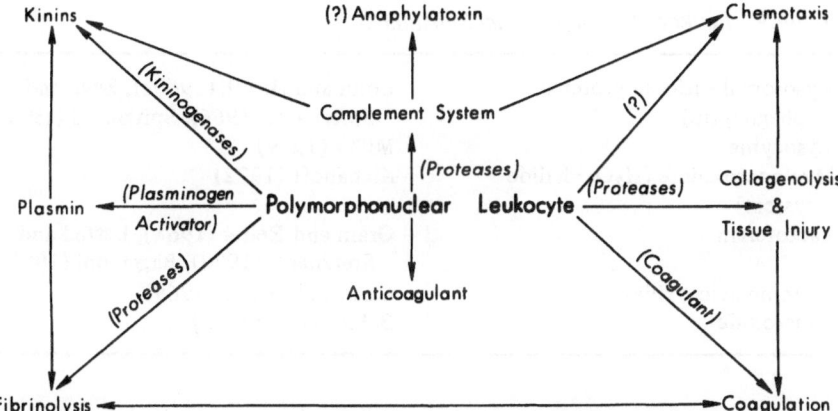

Fig. 2. Polymorphonuclear leukocytes and inflammatory mediator system interactions.

Three important factors regulate the activity of the leukokinin system. An acid pH is required, as this is necessary for leukokinin formation. Circulating substrate must be made available by activation of a plasma protease. And, finally, leukokininogenases must be released from within cells. Since each of these conditions may actually be met in sites of tissue injury, leukokinins may conceivably be biologically significant inflammatory mediators.

Although their significance remains unknown, two additional reports should be cited in this discussion of kinins. Hageman factor (Szpilman *et al.*, 1969) and activated Hageman factor (Prokopowicz *et al.*, 1972) have been isolated from human polymorphonuclear leukocytes obtained from pleural exudates.

Figure 2 depicts the role of the polymorphonuclear leukocyte in the generation of inflammatory mediators and illustrates some important interactions between mediator systems.

7. ANTIBACTERIAL SUBSTANCES

In this discussion of inflammatory materials contained within polymorphonuclear leukocytes, some mention of substances with antibacterial activity is warranted. Kanthack and Hardy (1894) were among the first investigators to observe the antibacterial action of leukocytic cytoplasmic granules and suggested that the granules contained unspecified substances toxic to bacterial cells. Several such substances have since been identified, and are listed in Table V (with appropriate references). Apart from the lysosomal cationic proteins, these antibacterial substances, or systems, have not been implicated in the mediation of tissue injury, except by virtue of the altered susceptibility to infection that results from their absence (see review by Klebanoff, 1971).

Table V. Leukocyte Antibacterial Substances

Lysosomal cationic proteins (phagocytin)	Cohn and Hirsch (1960a), Zeya and Spitznagel (1966), Spitznagel (1972)
Lysozyme	Miller (1969)
Myeloperoxidase (H_2O_2-halide system)	Klebanoff (1972)
Lactoferrin	Oram and Reiter (1968), Leffell and Spitznagel (1972), Baggiolini (1972)
D-amino acid oxidase	Cline and Lehrer (1969)
Superoxide	Babior et al. (1973)

8. CONCLUSIONS

Inflammatory reactions can be induced by a variety of offending agents. Regardless of etiology, however, tissue responses to injury are stereotyped and represent the combined effects of both humoral and cellular mediators. Although the origin, nature, and mode of action of many of the injurious substances contained within leukocytes have been elucidated, their precise roles in the production of these responses are not well understood. Intricate control mechanisms, as in other biological systems, which determine the initiation, propagation, and cessation of the inflammatory process are only beginning to be unraveled. It is not unreasonable to assume that during the next few years, as investigative efforts are directed toward these mechanisms, our understanding of the inflammatory process, and of the contributions made by leukocyte-derived substances to this process, will be greatly expanded.

9. REFERENCES

Ambache, N., Reynolds, M., and Whiting, J. M. C., 1963, Investigation of an active lipid in aqueous extracts of rabbit brain, and of some further hydroxyacids, *J. Physiol. (Lond.)* **166**:251.

Anderson, A. J., 1970, Lysosomal enzyme activity in rats with adjuvant-induced arthritis, *Ann. Rheum. Dis.* **29**:307.

Arya, D. V., Mannagh, J., and Irvine, A. R., Jr., 1972, Effect of lysosomes on cultured rabbit corneal cells, *Invest. Ophthalmol.* **11**:662.

Astrup, T., Henrichsen, J., and Kwaan, H. C., 1967, Protease content and fibrinolytic activity of human leukocytes, *Blood* **29**:134.

Avila, J. L., and Convit, J., 1973*a*, Studies on human polymorphonuclear leukocyte enzymes. I. Assay of acid hydrolases and other enzymes, *Biochim. Biophys. Acta* 293:397.

Avila, J. L., and Convit, J., 1973*b*, Studies on human polymorphonuclear leukocyte enzymes. II. Comparative study of the physical properties of primary and specific granules, *Biochim. Biophys. Acta* 293:409.

Avila, J. L., and Convit, J., 1973*c*, Heterogeneity of acid phosphatase activity in human polymorphonuclear leukocytes, *Clin. Chim. Acta* 44:21.

Babior, B. M., Kipnes, R. S., and Curnutte, J. T., 1973, Biological defense mechanisms: The production by leukocytes of superoxide, a potential bactericidal agent, *J. Clin. Invest.* 52:741.

Baggiolini, M., 1972, The enzymes of the granules of polymorphonuclear leukocytes and their functions, *Enzyme* 13:132.

Baggiolini, M., Hirsch, J. G., and deDuve, C., 1969, Resolution of granules from rabbit heterophil leukocytes into distinct populations by zonal sedimentation, *J. Cell Biol.* 40:529.

Baggiolini, M., Hirsch, J. G., and deDuve, C., 1970, Further biochemical and morphological studies of granule fractions from rabbit heterophil leukocytes, *J. Cell Biol.* 45:586.

Bainton, D. F., 1972, The origin, content and fate of PMN granules, in: *Phagocytic Mechanisms in Health and Disease* (R. C. Williams, Jr., and H. H. Fudenberg, eds.), pp. 123–136, Intercontinental Medical Book Corp., New York.

Bainton, D. F., 1973, Sequential degranulation of the two types of polymorphonuclear leukocyte granules during phagocytosis of microorganisms, *J. Cell Biol.* 58:249.

Bainton, D. F., and Farquhar, M. G., 1966, Origin of granules in polymorphonuclear leukocytes: Two types derived from opposite faces of the Golgi complex in developing granulocytes, *J. Cell Biol.* 28:277.

Bainton, D. F., and Farquhar, M. G., 1968*a*, Differences in enzyme content of azurophil and specific granules of polymorphonuclear leukocytes. II. Cytochemistry and electron microscopy of bone marrow cells, *J. Cell Biol.* 39:299.

Bainton, D. F., and Farquhar, M. G., 1968*b*, Differences in enzyme content of azurophil and specific granules of polymorphonuclear leukocytes. I. Histochemical staining of bone marrow smears, *J. Cell Biol.* 39:286.

Bainton, D. F., Ullyot, J. L., and Farquhar, M. G., 1971, The development of neutrophilic polymorphonuclear leukocytes in human bone marrow: Origin and content of azurophil and specific granules, *J. Exp. Med.* 134:907.

Barland, P., Novikoff, A. B., and Hamerman, D., 1964, Lysosomes in the synovial membrane in rheumatoid arthritis: A mechanism for cartilage erosion, *Trans. Assoc. Am. Physicians* 77:239.

Barnhart, M. I., 1965, Importance of neutrophilic leukocytes in the resolution of fibrin, *Fed. Proc.* 24:846.

Barnhart, M. I., 1968, Role of blood coagulation in acute inflammation, *Biochem. Pharmacol. Suppl.*, p. 205.

Barnhart, M. I., Quintana, C., Lenon, H. L., Bluhm, G. B., and Riddle, J. M., 1968, Proteases in inflammation, *Ann. N.Y. Acad. Sci.* 146:527.

Beeson, P. B., 1948, Temperature-elevating effect of a substance obtained from polymorphonuclear leukocytes, *J. Clin. Invest.* 27:524.

Bennett, I. L., Jr., and Beeson, P. B., 1953, Studies on the pathogenesis of fever. II. Characterization of fever-producing substances from polymorphonuclear leukocytes and from the fluid of sterile exudates, *J. Exp. Med.* 98:493.

Bodel, P., 1970, Studies on the mechanism of endogenous pyrogen production. I. Investigation of new protein synthesis in stimulated human blood leucocytes, *Yale J. Biol. Med.* 43:145.

Bodel, P., and Atkins, E., 1966, Human leukocyte pyrogen producing fever in rabbits, *Proc. Soc. Exp. Biol. Med.* 121:943.

Borel, J. F., Keller, H. U., and Sorkin, E., 1969, Studies on chemotaxis. XI. Effect on neutrophils of lysosomal and other subcellular fractions from leukocytes, *Int. Arch. Allergy Appl. Immunol.* 35:194.

Chang, J., Freer, R., Stella, R., and Greenbaum, L. M., 1972, Studies on leukokinins. II. Studies on the formation, partial amino acid sequence and chemical properties of leukokinins M and PMN, *Biochem. Pharmacol.* 21:3095.

Cline, M., 1973, Mechanism of acidification of the human leukocyte phagocytic vacuole, *Clin. Res.* 21:595.

Cline, M. J., and Lehrer, R. I., 1969, D-Amino-acid-linked antimicrobial system, *Proc. Natl. Acad. Sci.* 62:756.

Cochrane, C. G., and Aiken, B. S., 1966, Polymorphonuclear leukocytes in immunologic reactions: The destruction of vascular basement membrane *in vivo* and *in vitro, J. Exp. Med.* 124:733.

Cochrane, C. G., and Müller-Eberhard, H. J., 1968, The derivation of two distinct anaphyla-toxin activities from the third and fifth components of human complement, *J. Exp. Med.* 127:371.

Cochrane, C. G., Weigle, W. O., and Dixon, F. J., 1959, The role of polymorphonuclear leukocytes in the initiation and cessation of the Arthus vasculitis, *J. Exp. Med.* 110:481.

Cochrane, C. G., Unanue, E. R., and Dixon, F. J., 1965, A role for polymorphonuclear leukocytes and complement in nephrotoxic nephritis, *J. Exp. Med.* 122:99.

Coffey, J. W., and deDuve, C., 1968, Digestive activity of lysosomes. I. The digestion of proteins by extracts of rat liver lysosomes, *J. Biol. Chem.* 243:3255.

Cohn, Z. A., and Hirsch, J. G., 1960*a*, The isolation and properties of the specific cytoplasmic granules of rabbit polymorphonuclear leukocytes, *J. Exp. Med.* 112:983.

Cohn, Z. A., and Hirsch, J. G., 1960*b*, The influence of phagycotosis on the intracellular distribution of granule-associated components of polymorphonuclear leucocytes, *J. Exp. Med.* 112:1015.

Coppi, G., and Bonardi, G., 1968, Effect of two non-steroidal anti-inflammatory agents on alkaline and acid phosphatases of inflamed tissue, *J. Pharm. Pharmacol.* 20:661.

Cornely, H. P., 1966, Reversal of chemotaxis *in vitro* and chemotactic activity of leukocyte fractions, *Proc. Soc. Exp. Biol. Med.* 122:831.

Cranston, W. I., Goodale, F., Snell, E. S., and Wendt, F., 1956, The role of leukocytes in the initial action of bacterial pyrogens in man, *Clin. Sci.* 15:219.

Crowder, J. G., Martin, R. R., and White, A., 1969, Release of histamine and lysosomal enzymes by human leukocytes during phagocytosis of staphylococci, *J. Lab. Clin. Med.* 74:436.

Daems, W. T., 1968, On the fine structure of human neutrophilic leukocyte granules, *J. Ultrastruct. Res.* 24:343.

Davies, P., Rita, G. A., Krakauer, K., and Weissmann, G., 1971, Characterization of a neutral protease from lysosomes of rabbit polymorphonuclear leucocytes, *Biochem. J.* 123:559.

Davies, P., Krakauer, K., and Weissmann, G., 1972, Calf thymus histone as a substrate for neutral and acid proteases of leucocyte lysosomes and other proteolytic enzymes, *Anal. Biochem.* 45:428.

deDuve, C., Pressman, B. C., Gianetto, R., Wattiaux, R., and Appelmans, F., 1955, Tissue fractionation studies. 6. Intracellular distribution patterns of enzymes in rat liver tissue, *Biochem. J.* 60:604.

DeShazo, C. V., McGrade, M. T., Henson, P. M., and Cochrane, C. G., 1972, The effect of complement depletion on neutrophil migration in acute immunologic arthritis, *J. Immunol.* 108:1414.

Dingle, J. T., Poole, A. R., Lazarus, G. L., and Barrett, A. J., 1973, Immunoinhibition of intracellular protein digestion in macrophages, *J. Exp. Med.* 137:1124.

Edlow, D. W., and Sheldon, W. H., 1971, The pH of inflammatory exudates, *Proc. Soc. Exp. Biol. Med.* 137:1328.

Erdogan, G., 1968, The thromboplastic activity of white blood cells, *Blut.* 17:276.

Eriksson, S., 1964, Pulmonary emphysema and alpha$_1$-antitrypsin deficiency, *Acta Med. Scand.* 175:197.

Farquhar, M. G., Bainton, D. F., Baggiolini, M., and deDuve, C., 1972, Cytochemical localization of acid phosphatase activity in granule fractions from rabbit polymorphonuclear leukocytes, *J. Cell Biol.* 54:141.

Folds, J. D., Welsh, I. R. H., and Spitznagel, J. K., 1972, Neutral proteases confined to one class of lysosomes of human polymorphonuclear leukocytes, *Proc. Soc. Exp. Biol. Med.* 139:461.

Freer, R., Chang, J., and Greenbaum, L. M., 1972, Studies on leukokinins. III. Pharmacoligical activities of leukokinins M and PMN, *Biochem. Pharmacol.* 21:3107.

Galdston, M., Janoff, A., and Davis, A. L., 1973, Familial variation of leukocyte lysosomal protease and serum α_1-antitrypsin as determinants in chronic obstructive pulmonary disease, *Am. Rev. Resp. Dis.* 107:718.

Gans, H., 1963, Fibrinolytic properties of proteases derived from human, dog and rabbit leukocytes, *Thromb. Diath. Haemorrh.* 10:379.

Goetzl, E. J., and Austen, K. F., 1972, A neutrophil-immobilizing factor derived from human leukocytes. I. Generation and partial characterization, *J. Exp. Med.* 136:1564.

Goldstein, I. M., Wunschmann, B., Astrup, T., and Henderson, E. S., 1971, Effects of bacterial endotoxin on the fibrinolytic activity of normal human leukocytes, *Blood* 37:447.

Goldstein, I. M., Brai, M., Osler, A. G., and Weissman, G., 1973, Lysosomal enzyme release from human leukocytes: Mediation by the alternate pathway of complement activation, *J. Immunol.* 111:33.

Golub, E. S., and Spitznagel, J. K., 1966, The role of lysosomes in hypersensitivity reactions: Tissue damage by polymorphonuclear neutrophil lysosomes, *J. Immunol.* 95:1060.

Graham, H. T., Lowry, O. H., Wheelwright, F., Lenz, M. A., and Parish, H. H., Jr., 1955, Distribution of histamine among leukocytes and platelets, *Blood* 10:467.

Greenbaum, L. M., 1972, Leukocyte kininogenases and leukokinins from normal and malignant cells, *Am. J. Pathol.* 68:613.

Greenbaum, L. M., and Kim, K. S., 1967, The kinin-forming and kininase activities of rabbit polymorphonuclear leucocytes, *Brit. J. Pharmacol.* 29:238.

Greenbaum, L. M., Freer, R., Chang, J., Semente, G., and Yamafuji, K., 1969, PMN-kinin and kinin metabolizing enzymes in normal and malignant leucocytes, *Brit. J. Pharmacol.* 36:623.

Greenbaum, L. M., Prakash, A., and Semente, G., 1972, Studies on leukokininogen in plasma, *Fed. Proc.* 31:534.

Hahn, H. H., Cheuk, S. F., Dianne, C., Elfenbein, S., and Wood, W. B., Jr., 1970, Studies on the pathogenesis of fever, XIX. Localization of pyrogen in granulocytes, *J. Exp. Med.* 131:701.

Harris, E. D., Jr., DiBona, D. R., and Krane, S. M., 1969, Collagenases in human synovial fluid, *J. Clin. Invest.* 48:2104.

Hawiger, J., Collins, R. D., and Horn, R. G., 1969a, Precipitation of soluble fibrin monomer complexes by lysosomal protein fraction of polymorphonuclear leukocytes, *Proc. Soc. Exp. Biol. Med.* **131**:349.

Hawiger, J., Horn, R. G., Koenig, M. G., and Collins, R. D., 1969b, Activation and release of lysosomal enzymes from isolated leukocytic granules by liposomes: A proposed model for degranulation in polymorphonuclear leukocytes, *Yale J. Biol. Med.* **42**:57.

Hawiger, J., Hawiger, A., and Loenig, M. G., 1972, Activation of lysosomal enzymes in polymorphonuclear leukocyte granules: The role of phospholipid–protein interaction, *Yale J. Biol. Med.* **45**:42.

Henson, P. M., 1972, Pathologic mechanisms in neutrophil-mediated injury, *Am. J. Pathol.* **68**:593.

Herion, J. C., Spitznagel, J. K., Walker, R. I., and Zeya, H. I., 1966, Pyrogenicity of granulocyte lysosomes, *Am. J. Physiol.* **211**:693.

Hill, J. H., and Ward, P. A., 1969, C3 leukotactic factors produced by a tissue protease, *J. Exp. Med.* **130**:505.

Hill, J. H., and Ward, P. A., 1971, The phlogistic role of C3 leukotactic fragments in myocardial infarcts of rats, *J. Exp. Med.* **133**:885.

Hirsch, J. G., 1962, Cinemicrophotographic observations on granule lysis in polymorphonuclear leukocytes during phagocytosis, *J. Exp. Med.* **116**:827.

Hirsch, J. G., and Cohn, Z. A., 1960, Degranulation of polymorphonuclear leukocytes following phagocytosis of microorganisms, *J. Exp. Med.* **112**:1005.

Hirschhorn, R., and Weissmann, G., 1965, Isolation and properties of human leukocyte lysosomes *in vitro, Proc. Soc. Exp. Biol. Med.* **119**:36.

Hirschhorn, R., and Weissmann, G., 1967, Death of leucocytes due to ingestion of heterologous lysosomes, *Nature (Lond.)* **214**:892.

Horn, R. G., and Collins, R. D., 1968, Studies on the pathogenesis of the generalized Shwartzman reaction: The role of granulocytes, *Lab. Invest.* **18**:101.

Houck, J., and Chang, C., 1971, The chemotactic properties of the products of collagenolysis, *Proc. Soc. Exp. Biol. Med.* **138**:69.

Humphrey, J. H., 1955, The mechanism of the Arthus reaction. I. The role of polymorphonuclear leukocytes and other factors in reversed passive Arthus reactions in rabbits, *Brit. J. Exp. Pathol.* **36**:268.

Hurley, J. V., 1964, Substances promoting leukocyte emigration, *Ann. N.Y. Acad. Sci.* **116**:918.

Janoff, A., 1970, Mediators of tissue damage in leukocyte lysosomes. X. Further studies on human granulocyte elastase, *Lab. Invest.* **22**:228.

Janoff, A., 1972a, Human granulocyte elastase, *Am. J. Pathol.* **68**:579.

Janoff, A., 1972b, Inhibition of human granulocyte elastase by serum α_1-antitrypsin, *Am. Rev. Resp. Dis.* **105**:121.

Janoff, A., and Blondin, J., 1970, Depletion of cartilage matrix by a neutral protease fraction of human leukocyte lysosomes, *Proc. Soc. Exp. Biol. Med.* **135**:302.

Janoff, A., and Blondin, J., 1971, Inhibition of the elastase-like esterase in human leukocyte granules by human leukocyte cell sap, *Proc. Soc. Exp. Biol. Med.* **136**:1050.

Janoff, A., and Scherer, J., 1968, Mediators of inflammation in leukocyte lysosomes. IX. Elastinolytic activity in granules of human polymorphonuclear leukocytes, *J. Exp. Med.* **128**:1137.

Janoff, A., and Zeligs, J. D., 1968, Vascular injury and lysis of basement membrane *in vitro* by neutral protease of human leukocytes, *Science* **161**:702.

Janoff, A., and Zweifach, B. W., 1964, Adhesion and emigration of leukocytes produced by cationic proteins of lysosomes, *Science* **144**:1456.

Janoff, A., Rosenberg, R., and Galdston, M., 1971, Elastase-like, esteroprotease activity in human and rabbit alveolar macrophage granules, *Proc. Soc. Exp. Biol. Med.* 136:1054.

Janoff, A., Sandhaus, R. A., Hospelhorn, V. D., and Rosenberg, R., 1972, Digestion of lung proteins by human leukocyte granules *in vitro, Proc. Soc. Exp. Biol. Med.* 140:516.

Jensen, M. S., and Bainton, D. F., 1973, Temporal changes in pH within the phagocytic vacuole of the polymorphonuclear neutrophilic leukocyte, *J. Cell Biol.* 56:379.

Johanson, W. G., Jr., and Pierce, A. K., 1972, Effects of elastase, collagenase, and papain on structure and function of rat lungs *in vitro, J. Clin. Invest.* 51:288.

Jones, T. W., 1851, On the state of the blood and blood vessels in inflammation, *Guy's Hosp. Rep.* 7:1.

Kakinuma, K., 1970, Metabolic control and intracellular pH during phagocytosis by polymorphonuclear leucocytes, *J. Biochem. (Tokyo)* 68:177.

Kampschmidt, R. F., and Upchurch, H., 1969, Lowering of plasma iron concentration in the rat with leukocytic extracts, *Am. J. Physiol.* 216:1287.

Kampschmidt, R. F., and Upchurch, H. F., 1970, The effect of endogenous pyrogen on the plasma zinc concentration of the rat, *Proc. Soc. Exp. Biol. Med.* 134:1150.

Kang, A. H., Nagai, Y., Piez, K. A., and Gross, J., 1966, Studies on the structure of collagen using collagenolytic enzyme from tadpole, *Biochemistry* 5:509.

Kanthack, A. A., and Hardy, W. B., 1894, The morphology and distribution of the wandering cells of mammalia, *J. Physiol.* 17:81.

Kelly, M. T., Brashear, R. F., Martin, R. R., and White, A., 1971*a*, Histamine release in the dog after leukocyte lysate injection, *Infect. Immunity* 4:228.

Kelly, M. T., Martin, R. R., and White, A., 1971*b*, Mediators of histamine release from human platelets, lymphocytes, and granulocytes, 1971*b*, J. Clin. Invest. 50:1044.

Kerby, G. P., and Taylor, S. M., 1967, Enzymatic activity in human synovial fluid from rheumatoid and non-rheumatoid patients, *Proc. Soc. Exp. Biol. Med.* 126:865.

Klebanoff, S. J., 1971, Intraleukocytic microbicidal defects, *Ann. Rev. Med.* 22:39.

Klebanoff, S. J., 1972, The myeloperoxidase-mediated antimicrobial systems, in: *Phagocytic Mechanisms in Health and Disease* (R. C. Williams, Jr., and H. H. Fudenberg, eds.), pp. 3–21, Intercontinental Medical Book Corp., New York.

Kniker, W. T., and Cochrane, C. G., 1965, Pathogenic factors in vascular lesions of experimental serum sickness, *J. Exp. Med.* 122:83.

Kociba, G. J., and Griesemer, R. A., 1972, Disseminated intravascular coagulation induced with leukocyte procoagulant, *Am. J. Pathol.* 69:407.

Kociba, G. J., Loeb, W. F., and Wall, R. L., 1972, Development of procoagulant (tissue thromboplastin) activity in cultured leukocytes, *J. Lab. Clin. Med.* 79:778.

Koldajew, B., and Altschuler, M., 1930, Zur Frage über die aktive Reaktion der Exsudate bei chronischen und akuten Entzundungen, *Z. Immunitaetsforsch.* 69:18.

Kueppers, F., and Bearn, A. G., 1966, A possible experimental approach to the association of hereditary α_1-antitrypsin deficiency and pulmonary emphysema, *Proc. Soc. Exp. Biol. Med.* 121:*1207.*

Lack, C. H., 1963, Origin of blood fibrinolytic activity, *Lancet* 2:522.

Lack, C. H., and Ali, S. Y., 1964, Tissue activator of plasminogen, *Nature (Lond.)* 201:1030.

Lapresle, C., and Webb, T., 1962, The purification and properties of a proteolytic enzyme rabbit cathepsin E, and further studies on rabbit cathepsin D, *Biochem. J.* 84:455.

Lazarus, G. S., Brown, R. S., Daniels, J. R., and Fullmer, H. M., 1968*a*, Human granulocyte collagenase, *Science* 159:1483.

Lazarus, G. S., Daniels, J. R., Brown, R. S., Bladen, H. A., and Fullmer, H. M., 1968*b*, Degradation of collagen by a human granulocyte collagenolytic system, *J. Clin. Invest.* 47:2622.

Lazarus, G. S., Daniels, J. R., Lian, J., and Burleigh, M. C., 1972, Role of granulocyte collagenase in collagen degradation, *Am. J. Pathol.* 68:565.

Leffell, M. S., and Spitznagel, J. K., 1972, Association of lactoferrin with lysozyme in granules of human polymorphonuclear leukocytes, *Infect. Immunity* 6:761.

Lehman, M. A., Kream, J., and Brogna, D., 1964, Acid and alkaline phosphtase activity in the serum and synovial fluid of patients with arthritis, *J. Bone Joint Surg.* 46A:1732.

Lerner, R. G., Goldstein, R., and Cummings, G., 1971, Stimulation of human leukocyte thromboplastic activity by endotoxin, *Proc. Soc. Exp. Biol. Med.* 138:145.

Lieberman, J., and Gawad, M., 1971, Inhibitors and activators of leukocytic proteases in purulent sputum: Digestion of human lung and inhibition by alpha$_1$-antitrypsin, *J. Lab. Clin. Med.* 77:713.

Lieberman, J., and Kaneshiro, W., 1972, Inhibition of leukocytic elastase from purulent sputum by alpha$_1$-antitrypsin, *J. Lab. Clin. Med.* 80:88.

Luscombe, M., 1963, Acid phosphatase and catheptic activity in rheumatoid synovial tissue, *Nature (Lond.)* 197:1010.

Manaligod, J. R., Krakower, C. A., and Greenspon, S. A., 1969, Glomerular changes induced by extrarenal foci of inflammation and by polymorphonuclear cell lysates, *Am. J. Pathol.* 56:533.

Mandell, G. L., 1970, Intraphagosomal pH of human polymorphonuclear neutrophils, *Proc. Soc. Exp. Biol. Med.* 134:447.

Marco, V., Mass, B., Meranze, D. R., Weinbaum, G., and Kimbel, P., 1971, Induction of experimental emphysema in dogs using leukocyte homogenates, *Am. Rev. Resp. Dis.* 104:595.

Martin, H., and Roka, L., 1951, Beeinflussung der Blutgerinnung durch Leukocyten, *Klin. Wschr.* 29:510.

Mass, B., Ikeda, T., Meranze, D., Weinbaum, G., and Kimbel, P., 1972, Induction of experimental emphysema: Cellular and species specificity, *Am. Rev. Resp. Dis.* 106:385.

Matsuoka, M., Sakuragawa, N., and Shimaoka, M., 1969, Studies on fibrinolytic activities in normal human leukocytes, *Acta Med. Biol.* 16:91.

May, C. D., Levine, B., and Weissmann, G., 1970, Effects of compounds which inhibit antigenic release of histamine and phagocytic release of lysosomal enzymes on glucose utilization by leukocytes in humans, *Proc. Soc. Exp. Biol. Med.* 133:758.

McCutcheon, M., 1946, Chemotaxis in leukocytes, *Physiol. Rev.* 26:319.

McKay, D. G., 1972, Participation of components of the blood coagulation system in the inflammatory response, *Am. J. Pathol.* 67:181.

Melmon, K. L., and Cline, M. J., 1967, Interaction of plasma kinins and granulocytes, *Nature (Lond.)* 213:90.

Melmon, K. L., and Cline, J. J., 1968, The interaction of leukocytes and the kinin system, *Biochem. Pharmacol. Suppl.*, p. 271.

Menkin, V., 1938, Studies on inflammation; isolation of a factor concerned with increased capillary permeability in injury, *J. Exp. Med.* 67:129.

Metchnikoff, E., 1887, Sur la lutte des cellules de l'organisme contre l'invasion des microbes, *Ann. Inst. Pasteur* 1:321.

Miller, T. E., 1969, Killing and lysis of gram-negative bacteria through the synergistic effect of hydrogen peroxide, ascorbic acid, and lysozyme, *J. Bacteriol.* 98:949.

Moore, D. M., Cheuk, S. F., Morton, J. D., Berlin, R. D., and Wood, W. B., Jr., 1970, Studies on the pathogenesis of fever. XVIII. Activation of leukocytes for pyrogen production, *J. Exp. Med.* 131:179.

Moore, D. M., Murphy, P. A., Chesney, P. J., and Wood, W. B., Jr., 1973, Synthesis of endogenous pyrogen by rabbit leukocytes, *J. Exp. Med.* 137:1263.

Mounter, L. A., and Atiyeh, W., 1960, Proteases of human leukocytes, *Blood* 15:52.

Movat, H. Z., Uriuhara, T., Takeuchi, Y., and Macmorine, D. R. L., 1971a, The role of PMN-leukocyte lysosomes in tissue injury, inflammation and hypersensitivity. VII. Liberation of vascular permeability factors from PMN-leukocytes during "*in vitro*" phagocytosis, *Int. Arch. Allergy* 40:197.

Movat, H. Z., Macmorine, D. R. L., and Takeuchi, Y., 1971b, Role of PMN-leukocyte lysosomes in tissue injury, inflammation and hypersensitivity. VIII. Mode of action and properties of vascular permeability factors released by PMN-leukocytes during "*in vitro*" phagocytosis, *Int. Arch. Allergy* 40:218.

Nachman, R., Hirsch, J. G., and Baggiolini, M., 1972, Studies on isolated membranes of azurophil and specific granules from rabbit polymorphonuclear leukocytes, *J. Cell Biol.* 54:133.

Niemetz, J., 1972a, The role of protein synthesis on the generation of tissue factor activity by leukocytes, *Proc. Soc. Exp. Biol. Med.* 139:1276.

Niemetz, J., 1972b, Coagulant activity of leukocytes: Tissue factor activity, *J. Clin. Invest.* 51:307.

Niemetz, J., and Fani, K., 1971, Role of leukocytes in blood coagulation and the generalized Shwartzman reaction, *Nature New Biol.* 232:247.

Ohlsson, K., 1971, Neutral leucocyte proteases and elastase inhibited by plasma alpha$_1$-antitrypsin, *Scand. J. Clin. Lab. Invest.* 28:251.

Olsson, I., 1969, Isolation of human leukocyte granules using colloidal silica–polysaccharide density gradients, *Exp. Cell Res.* 54:325.

Opie, E. L., 1907, Experimental pleurisy: Resolution of a fibrinous exudate, *J. Exp. Med.* 9:391.

Opie, E. L., 1922, Intracellular digestion: The enzymes and anti-enzymes concerned, *Physiol. Rev.* 2:552.

Oram, J. D., and Reiter, B., 1968, Inhibition of bacteria by lactoferrin and other iron-chelating agents, *Biochim. Biophys. Acta* 170:351.

Orange, R. P., Valentine, M. D., and Austen, K. F., 1968, Antigen-induced release of slow reacting substance of anaphylaxis (SRS-A) in rats prepared with homologous antibody, *J. Exp. Med.* 127:767.

Parish, W. E., 1969, Effects of neutrophils on tissues: Experiments on the Arthus reaction, the flare phenomenon, and post-phagocytic release of lysosomal enzymes, *Brit. J. Dermatol.* 81:28 (Suppl. 3).

Pekarek, R. S., and Beisel, W. R., 1971, Characterization of the endogenous mediator(s) of serum zinc and iron depression during infection and other stresses, *Proc. Soc. Exp. Biol. Med.* 138:728.

Pekarek, R. S., Wannemacher, R. W., Jr., Chapple, F. E., III, Powanda, M. C., and Beisel, W. R., 1972, Further characterization and species specificity of leukocytic endogenous mediator (LEM), *Proc. Soc. Exp. Biol. Med.* 141:643.

Pekarek, R. S., Wannemacher, R. W., Jr., Powanda, M. C., and Beisel, W. R., 1973, Regulation of infection-induced alterations in host metabolism by a hormone-like mediator released from polymorphonuclear leukocytes, *Clin. Res.* 21:608.

Penniall, R., and Zeya, H. I., 1971, The effects of cationic proteins of rabbit polymorphonuclear leukocyte lysosomes on the respiratory activity of liver mitochondria, *Biochem. Biophys. Res. Commun.* 45:6.

Penniall, R., Holbrook, J. P., and Zeya, H. I., 1972, The inhibition of cytochrome oxidase by lysosomal cationic proteins of rabbit polymorphonuclear leukocytes, *Biochem. Biophys. Res. Commun.* 47:1271.

Phelps, P., 1969, Polymorphonuclear leukocyte motility *in vitro*. III. Possible release of a chemotactic substance after phagocytosis of urate crystals by polymorphonuclear leukocytes, *Arthritis Rheum.* **12**:197.

Poplawski, A., Prokopowicz, J., and Niewiarowski, S., 1969, Antiheparin activity in subcellular fractions of human granulocytes, *Thromb. Diath. Haemorrh.* **21**:170.

Prokopowicz, J., 1968, Distribution of fibrinolytic and proteolytic enzymes in subcellular fractions of human granulocytes, *Thromb. Diath. Haemorrh.* **19**:84.

Prokopowicz, J., and Stormorken, H., 1968, Fibrinolytic activity of leukocytes in smears of bone marrow and peripheral blood, *Scand. J. Haematol.* **5**:129.

Prokopowicz, J., Wolosowicz, N., and Szmitkowski, M., 1972, The purification of activated Hageman factor from human granulocytes, *Thromb. Diath. Haemorrh.* **27**:228.

Pruzansky, J. J., and Patterson, R., 1967, Subcellular distribution of histamine in human leucocytes, *Proc. Soc. Exp. Biol. Med.* **124**:56.

Pruzansky, J. J., and Patterson, R., 1970, Histamine in human leukocytes: Localization of histamine and beta-glucuronidase in human leucocytes, *Int. Arch. Allergy.* **37**:98.

Pushpakom, R. J., Hogg, J. C., Woolcock, A. J., Angus, A. E., Macklem, P. T., and Thurlbeck, W. M., 1970, Experimental papain-induced emphysema in dogs, *Am. Rev. Resp. Dis.* **102**:778.

Ranadive, N. S., and Cochrane, C. G., 1968, Isolation and characterization of permeability factors from rabbit neutrophils, *J. Exp. Med.* **128**:605.

Rapaport, S. I., and Hjort, P. F., 1967, The blood clotting properties of rabbit peritoneal leukocytes *in vitro*, *Thromb. Diath. Haemorrh.* **17**:222.

Riddle, J. M., and Barnhart, M. I., 1964, Ultrastructural study of fibrin dissolution via emigrated polymorphonuclear neutrophils, *Am. J. Pathol.* **45**:805.

Robertson, P. B., Ryel, R. B., Taylor, R. E., Shyn, K. W., and Fullmer, H. M., 1972, Collagenase: Localization in polymorphonuclear leukocyte granules in the rabbit, *Science* **177**:64.

Root, R. K., Nordlund, J. J., and Wolff, S. M., 1970, Factors affecting the quantitative production and assay of human leukocytic pyrogen, *J. Lab. Clin. Med.* **75**:679.

Rous, P., 1925, The relative reaction within living mammalian tissues. II. On the mobilization of acid material within cells, and the reaction as influenced by the cell state, *J. Exp. Med.* **41**:399.

Rulot, H., 1904, Intervention des leucocytes dans l'autolyse de la fibrine (Fibrinolyse de Dastre), *Arch. Int. Physiol.* **1**:152.

Saba, H., Roberts, H. R., and Herion, J. C., 1967, The anticoagulant activity of lysosomal cationic proteins from polymorphonuclear leukocytes, *J. Clin. Invest.* **46**:580.

Saba, H. I., Roberts, H. R., and Herion, J. C., 1968, Antiheparin activity of lysosomal cationic proteins from polymorphonuclear leukocytes, *Blood* **31**:369.

Saba, H. I., Herion, J. C., and Roberts, H. R., 1969, The effects of lysosomal cationic proteins from granulocytes on the coagulation and fibrinolytic systems, *Blood* **34**:835.

Saba, H. I., Herion, J. C., Walker, R. I., and Roberts, H. R., 1973, The procoagulant activity of granulocytes, *Proc. Soc. Exp. Biol. Med.* **142**:614.

Scherer, J., and Janoff, A., 1968, Mediators of inflammation in leukocyte lysosomes. VII. Observations on mast cell rupturing agents in different species, *Lab. Invest.* **18**:196.

Schumacher, H. R., and Agudelo, C. A., 1972, Intravascular degranulation of neutrophils: An important factor in inflammation? *Science* **175**:1139.

Seegers, W., and Janoff, A., 1966, Mediators of inflammation in leukocyte lysosomes. VI. Partial purification and characterization of a mast cell–rupturing component, *J. Exp. Med.* **124**:833.

Simpson, D., and Archer, G. T., 1967, Release of histamine from human basophils, *Blood* **29**:722.

Smith, C., and Hamerman, D., 1962, Acid phosphatase in human synovial fluid, *Arthritis Rheum.* 5:411.

Snyderman, R., Shin, H. S., and Dannenberg, A. M., Jr., 1972, Macrophage proteinase and inflammation: The production of chemotactic activity from the fifth component of complement by macrophage proteinase, *J. Immunol.* 109:896.

Spitznagel, J. K., 1972, Sorting out lysosomes and other cytoplasmic granules from polymorphs of rabbits and humans: A search for antibacterial factors, in: *Phagocytic Mechanisms in Health and Disease* (R. C. Williams, Jr., and H. H. Fudenberg, eds.), pp. 83–106, Intercontinental Medical Book Corp., New York.

Sprick, M. G., 1956, Phagocytosis of *M. tuberculosis* and *M. smegmatis* stained with indicator dyes, *Am. Rev. Tuberc. Pulm. Dis.* 74:552.

Statsny, P., and Ziff, M., 1970, Inhibitor of macrophage migration produced by polymorphonuclear leukocytes, *J. Reticuloendothel. Soc.* 7:140.

Stecher, V. J., and Sorkin, E., 1972, The chemotactic activity of fibrin lysis products, *Int. Arch. Allergy* 43:879.

Stetson, C. A., 1951, Similarities in the mechanisms determining the Arthus and Shwartzman phenomenon, *J. Exp. Med.* 94:347.

Stiles, M., and Fraenkel-Conrat, J., 1968, Subcellular distribution of human leukocytic cathepsins, *Blood* 32:119.

Szpilman, H., Prokopowicz, J., and Niewiarowski, S., 1969, Distribution of procoagulant activity in the subcellular fractions of human granulocytes, *Experientia (Basel)* 25:77.

Taubman, S. B., and Lepow, I. H., 1971, Cleavage of human C1$\bar{s}$ by human lysosomal enzymes, plasmin, and trypsin, *Immunochemistry* 8:951.

Taubman, S. B., Goldschmidt, P. R., and Lepow, I. H., 1970, Effects of lysosomal enzymes from human leukocytes on human complement components, *Fed. Proc.* 29:434.

Thomas, L., 1964, Possible role of leucocyte granules in the Shwartzman and Arthus reactions, *Proc. Soc. Exp. Biol. Med.* 115:235.

Wannemacher, R. W., Jr., DuPont, H. L., Pekarek, R. S., Powanda, M. D., Schwartz, A., Hornick, R. B., and Beisel, W. R., 1972*a*, An endogenous mediator of depression of amino acids and trace metals in serum during typhoid fever, *J. Infect. Dis.* 126:77.

Wannemacher, R. W., Jr., Pekarek, R. S., and Beisel, W. R., 1972*b*, Mediator of hepatic amino acid flux in infected rats, *Proc. Soc. Exp. Biol. Med.* 139:128.

Ward, P. A., 1967, A plasmin-split fragment of C'3 as a new chemotactic factor, *J. Exp. Med.* 126:189.

Ward, P. A., 1968, Chemotaxis of mononuclear cells, *J. Exp. Med.* 128:1201.

Ward, P. A., and Hill, H. J., 1970, C5 chemotactic fragments produced by an enzyme in lysosomal granules of neutrophils, *J. Immunol.* 104:535.

Ward, P. A., and Newman, L. J., 1969, A neutrophil chemotactic factor from human C5, *J. Immunol.* 102:93.

Wasi, S., Murray, R. K., Macmorine, D. R. L., and Movat, H. Z., 1966, The role of PMN-leucocyte lysosomes in tissue injury, inflammation and hypersensitivity. II. Studies on the proteolytic activity of PMN-leucocyte lysosomes of the rabbit, *Brit. J. Exp. Pathol.* 47:411.

Watanabe, I., Donahue, S., and Hoggatt, N., 1967, Method of electron microscopic studies of circulating human leukocytes and observations on their fine structure, *J. Ultrastruct. Res.* 20:366.

Weissmann, G., and Spilberg, I., 1968, Breakdown of cartilage protein polysaccharide by lysosomes, *Arthritis Rheum.* 9:162.

Weissmann, G., Spilberg, I., and Krakauer, K., 1969, Arthritis induced in rabbits by lysates of granulocyte lysosomes, *Arthritis Rheum.* 12:103.

Welsh, I. R. H., and Spitznagel, J. K., 1971, Distribution of lysosomal enzymes, cationic proteins, and bactericidal substances in subcellular fractions of human polymorphonuclear leukocytes, *Infect. Immunity* 4:97.

Wetzel, B. K., Spicer, S. S., and Horn, R. G., 1967, Fine structural localization of acid and alkaline phosphatases in cells of rabbit blood and bone marrow, *J. Histochem. Cytochem.* 15:311.

Wunschmann-Henderson, B., Horwitz, D. L., and Astrup, T., 1972, Release of plasminogen activator from viable leukocytes of man, baboon, dog and rabbit, *Proc. Soc. Exp. Biol. Med.* 141:634.

Zeya, H. I., and Spitznagel, J. K., 1966, Antimicrobial specificity of leukocyte lysosomal cationic proteins, *Science* 154:1049.

Zeya, H. I., and Spitznagel, J. K., 1968, Arginine-rich proteins of polymorphonuclear leukocyte lysosomes: Antimicrobial specificity and biochemical heterogeneity, *J. Exp. Med.* 127:927.

Zeya, H. I., and Spitznagel, J. K., 1971, Characterization of cationic protein-bearing granules of polymorphonuclear leukocytes, *Lab. Invest.* 24:229.

Zigmond, S. H., and Hirsch, J. G., 1973, Leukocyte locomotion and chemotaxis: New methods of evaluation, and demonstration of a cell-derived chemotactic factor, *J. Exp. Med.* 137:387.

Zucker-Franklin, D., and Hirsch, J. G., 1964, Electron microscope studies on the degranulation of rabbit peritoneal leukocytes during phagocytosis, *J. Exp. Med.* 120:569.

THE PLASMA KININ-FORMING SYSTEM

3

Jocelyn Spragg

1. INTRODUCTION

Because the nonapeptide bradykinin can elicit some of the phenomena associated with an inflammatory response, considerable attention has been devoted for some time to the plasma protein pathway leading to the generation of this mediator. Although earlier studies were devoted chiefly to *in vivo* models or to crude plasma fractions, recent work has focused on the use of highly purified proteins to examine the sequence and nature of their interactions in this pathway. From these investigations have come better physicochemical characterization of the components of the kinin-forming system, the recognition that several of these components in themselves have biological activity compatible with an inflammatory response, further examination of modes of activating the

Dr. Spragg is an Established Investigator of the American Heart Association, Inc. The author's work described herein was done during the tenure of a postdoctoral fellowship from the Arthritis Foundation and was supported by Grants AI-07722, AM-05577, and RR-05669 from the National Institutes of Health and by a grant from the John A. Hartford Foundation, Inc.

JOCELYN SPRAGG Department of Medicine, Harvard Medical School, and Department of Medicine, Robert B. Brigham Hospital, Boston, Massachusetts kinin-forming sequence, and an increased understanding of the multiplicity of interactions of this sequence with other plasma systems implicated in inflammation. This chapter will discuss information in these areas, with a focus on studies using human material.

2. BIOLOGICAL ACTIVITIES OF COMPONENTS AND THEIR INHIBITION

The pathway leading to the formation of bradykinin is initiated by the activation of Hageman factor and results in the conversion of a series of proenzymes to their active forms with the resultant generation of several biological activities in addition to those of bradykinin. Herein are described this pathway as it is presently understood and the actions of its components.

2.1. The Several Forms of Hageman Factor; PF/dil

Once activated (see Section 6.1), Hageman factor (clotting factor XII) acts on three plasma proenzymes to convert them to their active forms (Fig. 1). Pre-plasma thromboplastin antecedent (pre-PTA), or clotting factor XI, is activated to initiate the intrinsic coagulation mechanism (Ratnoff *et al.*, 1961); plasminogen proactivator is converted to plasminogen activator, leading to

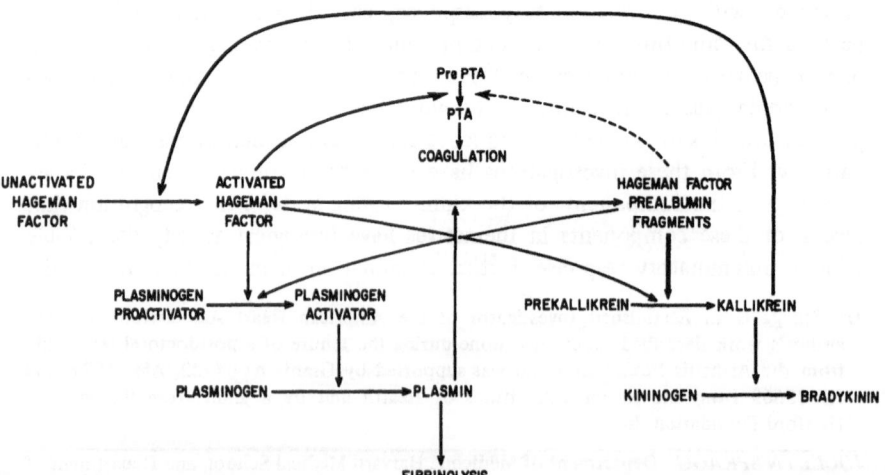

Fig. 1. Schematic representation of the plasma kinin-forming pathway.

plasmin formation (Kaplan and Austen, 1972); and prekallikrein is converted to kallikrein, leading to kinin generation (Kaplan and Austen, 1971). The active forms of PTA, plasmin, and kallikrein (Revak *et al.*, 1973; Cochrane *et al.*, 1972*a*, 1973) further activate Hageman factor, thus providing positive feedback loops in this system; the last of these enzymes is held to be 3–10 times more active on a molar basis than the first two (Cochrane *et al.*, 1973).

Active Hageman factor is digested by plasmin to intermediate-size fragments and then to Hageman factor prealbumin fragments (Fig. 1) (Kaplan and Austen, 1971; Kaplan *et al.*, 1971), which have been most extensively studied (Kaplan and Austen, 1972; Schreiber *et al.*, 1973*a,b*). They act on the same precursor enzymes as the parent Hageman factor; however, in the fluid phase, activation of pre-PTA occurs more rapidly with intact activated Hageman factor than with the prealbumin fragments, whereas activation of prekallikrein proceeds more effectively with the fragments than with the intact parent molecule (Kaplan and Austen, 1971). Thus by fragmenting active Hageman factor, plasmin diverts the sequence from activation of clotting to generation of kinin. Following the recognition that the prealbumin prekallikrein activator is a fragment of activated Hageman factor (Kaplan and Austen, 1970), similar prealbumin activities isolated at the same time in the rabbit (prokininogenase activator, Wuepper *et al.*, 1970), guinea pig (Treloar and Movat, 1970), and man (Movat *et al.*, 1971; Wuepper and Cochrane, 1971) were also shown to be derived from Hageman factor (Cochrane and Wuepper, 1971*b*; Soltay *et al.*, 1971).

It seems likely that forms of activated Hageman factor are now functionally synonymous with the activity termed "PF/dil." PF/dil refers to the ability to increase vascular permeability after intradermal injection of guinea pigs with human or guinea pig plasma that has been diluted a hundredfold with normal saline and allowed to stand in contact with glass for 1 h (MacKay *et al.*, 1953; Stewart and Bliss, 1957). As this function could not be generated in Hageman factor deficient plasma (Ratnoff and Miles, 1964) and could be released from fresh but not heat-inactivated plasma, it was thought to act before kallikrein (Mason and Miles, 1962). DEAE chromatography of serum revealed two regions with this activity, a γ-globulin fraction containing kallikrein and a β-globulin fraction whose activity was attributed to PF/dil (Kagan *et al.* 1963). The evidence that PF/dil corresponds to forms of activated Hageman factor includes (a) the chromatographic isolation of certain of the Hageman factor fragments from the β-region on DEAE-cellulose chromatography of serum (Kaplan and Austen, 1970), (b) the failure to generate PF/dil from plasma deficient in Hageman factor (Ratnoff and Miles, 1964) or prekallikrein (Wuepper, 1972) until reconstitution with the missing factor (Weiss *et al.*, 1973), and (c) the removal of PF/dil activity generated in the classical fashion with a monospecific antibody to Hageman factor (Johnston *et al.*, 1974). Although prekallikrein is required for the formation of PF/dil activity (Wuepper, 1972), exposure of diluted, glass-treated plasma to a prekallikrein immunoadsorbent failed to remove PF/dil (Johnston *et al.*, 1974).

2.2. Plasminogen Activator

Highly purified plasminogen activator has been shown to convert plasminogen to plasmin (Fig. 1) without a requirement for streptokinase (Kaplan and Austen, 1972) and to be chemotactic for human polymorphonuclear leukocytes (Kaplan *et al.*, 1973). This latter activity was shown to be distinct from the chemotactic activity of kallikrein not only by the use of highly purified reagents but also by its identification in Fletcher trait plasma which is congenitally deficient in prekallikrein (Kaplan *et al.*, 1973), and its inhibition by α_2-macroglobulin, but not by the inhibitor of the first component of complement (CĪINH) (Goetzl and Austen, 1974). The inhibition of both functions of plasminogen activator by diisopropyl fluorophosphate (DFP) indicates a requirement for an active enzymatic site (Kaplan and Austen, 1972; Kaplan *et al.*, 1973).

A plasma factor restoring the kaolin-induced fibrinolytic activity known to be deficient in Hageman trait plasma has been designated the Hageman factor cofactor (Ogston *et al.*, 1969, 1971). Because of similarities in activation, function, chromatographic properties, and lack of inhibition by CĪINH, Hageman factor cofactor may represent an aggregated or complexed form of the plasminogen (pro)activator (Kaplan and Austen, 1972).

2.3. Plasmin

In addition to further activating Hageman factor (Cochrane *et al.*, 1972a) and converting active Hageman factor to its fragments (Fig. 1) (Kaplan and Austen, 1971; Burrowes *et al.*, 1971) as noted above, plasmin converts the first component of complement to an active enzymatic form (Ratnoff and Naff, 1967) and releases anaphylatoxin (C3a) from the third component of complement (Ward, 1967), thereby generating biologically active molecules of the complement system by mechanisms independent of immunological activation (Ruddy, this volume, Chapter 4). The action of plasmin on fibrinogen produces two intermediate digestion products with molecular weights of 240,000 (fragment X) and 155,000 (fragment Y) shown to have anticoagulant activity (Marder and Shulman, 1969). Using canine reagents, it has been shown that the later-stage degradation products produced by plasmin, factors D (85,000 mol wt) and E (50,000 mol wt), have, respectively, granulocyte chemotactic activity *in vivo* and the ability to enhance vascular permeability in skin (Barnhart *et al.*,

1971). Whether a factor chemotactic for neutrophils *in vitro* is derived from the action of plasmin on human fibrin (but not on fibrinogen) (Stecher and Sorkin, 1972) is unclear in light of a recent report demonstrating that the action of thrombin on fibrinogen to convert it to fibrin produces a chemotactic factor and that synthetic fibrinopeptide B is chemotactic (Kay *et al.*, 1973).

The early views that plasmin directly cleaved kininogen (Lewis, 1958; Ratnoff, 1965) or activated prekallikrein (Seidel *et al.*, 1969; Vogt, 1964) have not been substantiated by studies with highly purified reagents, which show that plasmin has no direct effect on prekallikrein (Kaplan and Austen, 1971) and directly cleaves kininogen only at high concentrations (Seidel *et al.*, 1971). Recent evidence indicates that the role of plasmin in kinin generation is at the level of Hageman factor cleavage (Kaplan and Austen, 1971; Burrowes *et al.*, 1971; Kaplan *et al.*, 1971).

2.4. Kallikrein

Plasma kallikrein (Fig. 1) cleaves a plasma substrate, kininogen, to release the nonapeptide, bradykinin (Webster and Pierce, 1963). Recent evidence indicating that the bradykinin sequence is located internally in kininogen (see Section 3.6) would suggest that kallikrein cleaves kininogen at two points or that another enzyme is required to release bradykinin from its substrate. Kallikrein also demonstrates chemotaxis for polymorphonuclear leukocytes, which, like the chemotactic activity of plasminogen activator, is inhibitable by DFP (Kaplan *et al.*, 1972). As noted above (Section 2.1), a third function is the reciprocal activation of Hageman factor (Cochrane *et al.*, 1972*a,b*).

2.5. Bradykinin

Because the sequence of isolated native bradykinin was determined some years ago (Boissonnas *et al.*, 1960; Elliott *et al.*, 1960) and synthetic bradykinin has been available for close to a decade (Merrifield, 1964), considerable attention has been devoted to the physiological and pharmacological actions of this nonapeptide.* Bradykinin is an extremely potent hypotensive agent, producing in millimicrogram quantities both increased vascular permeability and vasodilatation. It stimulates a variety of smooth muscle preparations in picogram and millimicrogram doses and is a potent elicitor of pain. Earlier work demonstrating leukocyte sticking after the introduction of Hageman factor into rabbit ear

---

* For extensive reviews of the actions of bradykinin, see Erdös (1966) and relevant chapters in Erdös (1970).

chambers (Graham *et al.*, 1965) can probably be attributed to the chemotactic activities of kallikrein and plasminogen activator (see Sections 2.2 and 2.4) rather than to bradykinin generation. Recent evidence showed that bradykinin in doses of 0.01–1.0 µg was not chemotactic *in vitro* for either eosinophils or neutrophils (Kaplan *et al.*, 1972).

2.6. Inhibitors of Enzymes in the Kinin-Forming System

Of the identified plasma inhibitors of proteolytic enzymes, three have been extensively examined with regard to their ability to inhibit the enzymes in the kinin-forming sequence. These observations have been compiled qualitatively in Table I.

The inhibitor of the activated first component of complement ($\overline{\text{CI}}$INH) has been shown to inhibit the coagulation function of activated Hageman factor (Forbes *et al.*, 1970) as well as the action of Hageman factor fragments on their three proenzyme substrates (Schreiber *et al.*, 1973*a*) and on benzoyl arginine ethyl ester (Özge-Anwar *et al.*, 1972). After incubation of Hageman factor fragments with $\overline{\text{CI}}$INH, the fragments were not demonstrable either functionally or electrophoretically, while the $\overline{\text{CI}}$INH titer was undiminished as assessed by effective molecule titration, suggesting either consumption of Hageman factor by $\overline{\text{CI}}$INH or the presence of two inhibitory sites (Schreiber *et al.*, 1973*a*). Neither α_2-macroglobulin (α_2-M) nor α_1-antitrypsin (α_1-AT) was capable of inhibiting the activity of Hageman factor fragments on their three proenzyme substrates (Schreiber *et al.*, 1973*b*).

After activation, these three enzymes are inhibited as follows: $\overline{\text{CI}}$INH inhibits the esterase activity of kallikrein (Kagan, 1964), its action on kininogen (Gigli *et al.*, 1970; McConnell, 1972; Schreiber *et al.*, 1973*a*), and its chemotactic activity toward polymorphonuclear leukocytes (Goetzl and Austen, 1973). In contrast to its inhibition of Hageman factor fragments, $\overline{\text{CI}}$INH consumption appears to be associated with the inhibition of both plasma kallikrein (Gilgi *et al.*, 1970; Schreiber *et al.*, 1973*a*) and $\overline{\text{CI}}$ esterase (Gigli *et al.*, 1968; Forbes *et al.*, 1970). α_2-M inhibits the kinin-generating (Harpel, 1970; McConnell, 1972; Schreiber *et al.*, 1973*b*) and chemotactic (Goetzl and Austen, 1973) functions of kallikrein. Earlier reports that α_1-AT inhibited kallikrein (Fritz *et al.*, 1972; McConnell, 1972) have not been confirmed (Schreiber *et al.*, 1973*b*). The ability of plasminogen activator to convert plasminogen to plasmin is inhibited by α_2-M (Schreiber *et al.*, 1973*b*), as is its chemotactic activity toward polymorphonuclear leukocytes (Goetzl and Austen, 1973); neither activity is inhibited by $\overline{\text{CI}}$INH or α_1-AT (Schreiber *et al.*, 1973*b*; Kaplan and Austen, 1972; E. J. Goetzl, personal communication). PTA is inhibited by $\overline{\text{CI}}$INH (Forbes *et al.*, 1970) as well as by another plasma protein with molecular weight of 65,000 (Amir *et al.*, 1972), but not by α_2-M (Harpel, 1971).

Table I. Inhibitors of Enzymes in the Kinin-Forming System[a]

Enzyme	Reaction	Inhibited by		
		CĪNH	α₁-AT	α₂-M
Activated Hageman factor	Pre-PTA→PTA	+	+	+
	Plasminogen proactivator→plasminogen activator			
	Prekallikrein→kallikrein			
Hageman factor fragments	Pre-PTA→PTA	+	o	o
	Plasminogen proactivator→plasminogen activator	+	o	o
	Prekallikrein→kallikrein	+	o	o
Plasminogen activator	Plasminogen→plasmin	o	o	+
	Chemotaxis	o	o	+
Plasma kallikrein	Kininogen→kinin	+	o	+
	Chemotaxis	+	o	+
PTA	Coagulation	+	+	0
Plasmin	Fibrinolysis	+	+	+

[a] For references, see text.

The fibrinolytic activity of plasmin is inhibited by $\overline{\text{CI}}$INH (Ratnoff *et al.*, 1969), by α_1-AT (Norman and Hill, 1958), and, on a molar basis, most effectively by α_2-M (Schreiber *et al.*, 1973*b*).

Thus the enzymes of the kinin-forming system can be controlled at several points along the pathway to the generation of biologically active molecules. A further point of control is the rapid destruction of bradykinin by two kininases, an arginine carboxypeptidase identified with the anaphylatoxin inactivator and a dipeptidase thought to be the same as the angiotensin I converting enzyme (see Section 3.7).

3. PREPARATION AND PHYSICOCHEMICAL CHARACTERIZATION OF COMPONENTS

The recent attention to purification and characterization of components of the kinin-forming system has led to increased understanding of the nature of their interactions and interrelationships with other plasma systems. Hence the general purification methodology and the physicochemical data so far obtained are presented to permit comparison with proteins of other plasma systems.

3.1. Precursor and Active Hageman Factor

Fractionation of fresh human plasma on quarternary aminoethyl (QAE) Sephadex at pH 8 yielded unactivated (i.e., precursor) Hageman factor early in the β-region as assessed by its ability on interaction with kaolin to correct the clotting deficiency of Hageman factor deficient plasma. This pooled peak, when applied to sulfoethyl (SE) Sephadex at pH 6 eluted as a broad peak between 0.25 and 0.35 M NaCl. After purification by QAE-, SE-, and G100-Sephadex passage (Kaplan *et al.*, 1971), the preparation containing unactivated Hageman factor (mol wt 110,000 by gel filtration, Table II) revealed two bands on disc gel electrophoresis: one in the γ-region corresponding to unactivated Hageman factor when assayed functionally and the other antigenically identical to transferrin. Acrylamide gel isoelectric focusing (Righetti and Drysdale, 1971) of the same preparation showed a series of double bands corresponding to the region of functional activity, with an isoelectric point ranging from pH 5.8 to 7.5 and peaking between pH 6.1 and 6.5 (Table II). Unactivated Hageman factor, eluted from the focusing gels between pH 6.4 and 7.2, was free of contaminants as demonstrated by reexamination on disc gel electrophoresis (Spragg *et al.*, 1973).

Unactivated Hageman factor, obtained from plasma by QAE-Sephadex chromatography and G100 gel filtration, was then chromatographed on car-

Table II. Physicochemical Characteristics of Components of the Human Plasma Kinin-Forming System

Component	Mol wt[a]	pI[b]	Mobility	Contaminant
Unactivated Hageman factor	110,000	5.8–7.5[c]	γ_1	None
Activated Hageman factor	110,000	5.8–7.5	γ_1	Trace IgG
Hageman factor prealbumin fragments	30,000–35,000	4.4–4.6	Prealbumin	None
Plasminogen proactivator	100,000	8.7–9.0[d]	γ_2	None
Plasminogen activator	100,000	8.6–8.9[d]	γ_2	Trace IgG
Plasminogen	80,000[e]	6.3–8.6	β	None
Plasmin	75,400[e]	6.1–8.4[f]	β	–
Prekallikrein	127,000	8.5–8.9[d]	γ_2	None
Kallikrein	108,000	8.5–8.9[d]	γ_2	Trace IgG
Pre-PTA	175,000	8.9–9.2[d]	γ_2	None
PTA	170,000	8.9–9.2[d]	γ_2	Trace IgG
Kininogen	70,000	4.5–4.7	Pretransferrin	Albumin

[a]Molecular weights were determined by Sephadex gel filtration characteristics, with the exception of kininogen, which was calculated from values for Stokes' radius, sedimentation coefficient, and partial specific volume (Spragg and Austen, 1971).
[b]Determined using analytical acrylamide gels (Righetti and Drysdale, 1971).
[c]Located by clotting assay after kaolin activation; peak activity was found between pH 6.1 and 6.5.
[d]Peak activities; plasminogen proactivator, 8.90; plasminogen activator, 8.8; prekallikrein, 8.75; kallikrein, 8.70; pre-PTA, 9.10; and PTA, 9.10.
[e]Barlow et al. (1969) by analytical ultracentrifugation.
[f]Determined after activation of plasminogen with streptokinase.

boxymethyl (CM) cellulose at pH 6, where it eluted between 0.22 and 0.30 M NaCl. Contact with CM-cellulose activated Hageman factor, in that the eluate corrected the clotting deficiency of Hageman-deficient plasma without a requirement for activation by kaolin (Kaplan and Austen, 1970). After these three purification steps, activated Hageman factor (mol wt 110,000 by Sephadex gel filtration) was shown on disc gel electrophoresis and by isoelectric focusing to have the same mobility and pI as unactivated Hageman factor (Table II). On focusing, it displayed the same double-banding pattern as unactivated Hageman factor (Spragg et al., 1973).

Cochrane and Wuepper (1971b) have found the molecular weight of unactivated Hageman factor to be 110,000–120,000 by G200 gel filtration and 90,000 by SDS gel electrophoresis (Cochrane et al., 1972b). For unactivated Hageman factor, Soltay et al. (1971) observed a molecular weight of 86,000 by sucrose density gradient ultracentrifugation and an isoelectric point of 5.0–5.5

in sucrose columns; their molecular weight for activated Hageman factor was 118,000 by gel filtration.

3.2. Hageman Factor Fragments

When blood was allowed to clot in glass, thereby activating Hageman factor, and chromatographed on diethylaminoethyl (DEAE) cellulose at pH 7.8, four peaks capable of correcting the clotting defect of Hageman-deficient plasma and converting partially purified prekallikrein to kallikrein were found (Kaplan and Austen, 1970). The converting activities were attributed to activated Hageman factor and a series of degradation products of progressively smaller size and greater net negative charge as assessed by Sephadex G100 gel filtration and disc gel electrophoresis. The size, electrophoretic mobility, and isoelectric point of these peaks were 110,000, γ1, and pH 6.1–6.5 (Hageman factor); 90,000, β, and pH 4.9–5.1; 60,000 and α; 30,000–35,000, prealbumin, and pH 4.4–4.6 (Kaplan et al., 1971; Kaplan and Austen, 1971).

The purification of an intermediate-size Hageman factor fragment was accomplished by collection of the plasma fraction eluted from QAE-Sephadex with 0.04 M NaCl, activation in glass, rechromatography on QAE-Sephadex, and filtration on Sephadex G100, where it eluted at a molecular weight of 80,000. A β-mobility was seen on disc gel electrophoresis (Schreiber et al., 1973a). The smallest fragments, designated "Hageman factor prealbumin fragments," were isolated from serum by DEAE-cellulose chromatography at pH 7.8, Sephadex G100 gel filtration, and CM-cellulose chromatography at pH 6.0, where they appeared with the effluent, and elution from disc gels after electrophoresis at pH 9.3 (Kaplan and Austen, 1970). Alternatively, unactivated Hageman factor was partially separated and the fragments were then generated and isolated. The effluent from DE52 chromatography of plasma with 0.05 M PO_4 buffer, known to contain unactivated Hageman factor, plasminogen proactivator, prekallikrein, and plasminogen, was pooled, activated by stirring in glass and chromatographed on QAE-, G100-, and SE-Sephadex (Kaplan et al., 1971). The fragments were identified functionally as a series of two to four prealbumin bands on disc gel electrophoresis and on isoelectric focusing as two to four bands isoelectric between pH 4.4 and 4.6 (Spragg et al., 1973) (Table II). The preparative procedure has been recently modified in that the plasma fraction eluted from QAE-Sephadex with 0.6 M NaCl at pH 8.0 was activated by stirring in glass, rechromatographed on QAE-Sephadex, and filtered on Sephadex G100 (Schreiber et al., 1973a).

Hageman factor fragments with size and charge like those of prealbumin fragments are also obtained on reduction and alkylation of ^{125}I-labeled intact Hageman factor, leading to the proposal that Hageman factor is composed of three polypeptide chains held together by disulfide bonds located at the ends of the chains (Cochrane *et al.*, 1972*b*). Recent data suggest that this structure may represent a postsynthetic modification of Hageman factor (readily obtainable in the rabbit) and that the intact molecule in both rabbit and man consists of a single polypeptide chain (C. G. Cochrane, personal communication).

3.3. Plasminogen Proactivator and Activator

The initial effluent obtained from the QAE-Sephadex chromatography of plasma at pH 8.0 containing IgG, plasminogen proactivator, prekallikrein, and unactivated PTA was pooled, concentrated, and chromatographed on SE-Sephadex at pH 6.0 and then filtered twice on Sephadex G150 and passed over an anti-IgG immunoadsorbant. The plasminogen proactivator was located functionally by activation with purified Hageman factor or Hageman factor fragments and assessment of its resultant capacity to convert purified plasminogen to plasmin (Kaplan and Austen, 1972). Plasminogen proactivator was shown by Sephadex G150 gel filtration to have a molecular weight of 100,000. Its mobility on disc gel electrophoresis was γ_2, and its isoelectric point determined functionally was 8.9 (Kaplan and Austen, 1972) (Table II).

Plasminogen activator, purified from serum by three chromatographic steps, when examined by the methods used for the precursor, gave the same results for molecular weight and mobility, and showed a slightly more acidic isoelectric point (Spragg *et al.*, 1973) (Table II).

3.4. Plasminogen and Plasmin

Plasminogen has been prepared from plasma fraction $III_{2,3}$ paste by isoelectric precipitation, chromatography on DEAE-Sephadex at pH 9.0, and filtration through G100 at the same pH (Robbins *et al.*, 1965). After activation of the plasma paste with streptokinase or urokinase, plasmin was isolated by the same procedure (Robbins *et al.*, 1965). A method of separating plasminogen directly from fresh plasma by adsorption on lysine–Sepharose and elution with ε-amino-caproic acid at pH 7.4 avoids the denaturing conditions of the previous procedure (Deutsch and Mertz, 1970); plasmin is obtained by activation of the eluted plasminogen with streptokinase. The physicochemical characteristics of plasminogen and plasmin are presented in Table II.

3.5. Prekallikrein and Kallikrein

The initial effluent in the QAE-Sephadex chromatography of plasma at pH 8.0 was applied to SE-Sephadex at pH 6.0, where prekallikrein eluted at 0.12 M

NaCl. It was located functionally by activation with Hageman factor or its fragments, and the resultant kallikrein was measured for its ability to release kinin from heat-inactivated plasma or partially purified kininogen (Kaplan *et al.*, 1971). After two chromatographic steps, gel filtration, and elution from disc gels, prekallikrein was contaminated only by small quantities of γ-globulin. This preparation was shown by gel filtration and functional analysis to have a molecular weight of 127,000; its mobility on disc gel electrophoresis was γ_2 and its isoelectric point was between 8.5 and 8.9 (Kaplan *et al.*, 1972) (Table II).

The effluent obtained from the DEAE-cellulose chromatography of serum at pH 8.0, containing kallikrein, PTA, IgG, and plasminogen activator, was fractionated by Sephadex G150 filtration. Further purification by CM-cellulose chromatography or SE-Sephadex chromatography resulted in low yields of the active enzyme. Therefore, when highly purified material was required it was prepared by activating purified prekallikrein with Hageman factor fragments. Active kallikrein, prepared in either manner, had a disc gel mobility and isoelectric point similar to those of prekallikrein, although on Sephadex gel filtration its molecular weight was 108,000 (Kaplan *et al.*, 1971).

Both human plasma prekallikrein and kallikrein were reported by Wuepper and Cochrane (1972) to have a molecular weight of 107,000 by SDS gel electrophoresis and an isoelectric point of 7.7 in sucrose columns. Movat *et al.* (1971) showed for kallikrein a molecular weight of 90,000–100,000 by gel filtration and a pI of 7.2–8.8 in sucrose columns. Colman *et al.* (1969) had earlier ascribed to kallikrein a molecular weight of about 100,000 by gel filtration and a γ-mobility on disc gel electrophoresis.

3.6. Kininogen

Kininogen isolated from fresh human plasma by DE52 chromatography and G100 gel filtration had a molecular weight of 70,000 as calculated from Stokes' radius, sedimentation coefficient, and partial specific volume (Table II) (Spragg and Austen, 1971), and was further purified electrophoretically. Using kininogen recovered from disc gel electrophoresis, where it migrated as a pretransferrin, the molecular weight in 10% SDS gels was 79,000 (Spragg *et al.*, 1973). Its isoelectric point determined both functionally and antigenically was 4.5–4.7 (Spragg and Austen, 1971) (Table II). Because of the reported functional and physicochemical diversity of human plasma kininogens (see below), this molecule was examined under various modifying conditions. Certain alterations or prolongation of the preparative procedures resulted in a retardation in the disc gel mobility of kininogen; that this was due to aggregation was supported by the observation that the original mobility was restored in disc gels run in 8 M urea. Treatment of kininogen with neuraminidase also retarded its disc gel mobility without diminishing its biological function. Either alterations in the preparative procedure or neuraminidase treatment shifted the isoelectric point of kininogen from pH 4.5–4.7 to 5.4–5.5 (Spragg and Austen, 1971).

The partial purification and characterization of human plasma substrates susceptible to kininogen-cleaving enzymes have been undertaken by several groups and reviewed (Pierce, 1968; Rocha e Silva, 1970; Webster, 1969). Two kininogens, separable by hydroxylapatite chromatography and having similar molecular weights (50,000) (Pierce, 1968) but different electrophoretic mobilities and susceptibility to inactivation of the kinin moiety by carboxypeptidase B, have been described (Pierce and Webster, 1966). Partially purified kininogens of molecular weight 197,000, a β-mobility, and $S_{20,\omega}$ = 7.68 and of molecular weight 57,000, an α_1-mobility, and $S_{20,\omega}$ = 3.65 (Jacobsen and Kriz, 1967) have been examined with regard to their enzyme susceptibilities. The former reacted rapidly with a plasma pseudoglobulin preparation used as a source of plasma kallikrein, and both reacted well with human saliva used as a source of glandular kallikrein (Jacobsen, 1966), leading to the suggestion that kininogens of molecular weight 200,000 represent the only substrate for plasma kallikrein (Webster, 1969). Subsequently, two kininogens, one having a molecular weight slightly less than that of IgG by gel filtration and with $S_{20,\omega}$ = 4.2 and the other with a molecular weight slightly greater than that of albumin and $S_{20,\omega}$ = 3.8, have been described; the former was reported to be the better substrate for plasma kallikrein (Habal and Movat, 1972). However, as noted above, kininogen with an apparent molecular weight of greater than 100,000 by gel filtration and a β-mobility on disc gel electrophoresis has been shown to exhibit a pretransferrin mobility in the presence of 8 M urea (Spragg and Austen, 1971).

Using a rapid, single-step separation, two kininogen-containing fractions have been identified on DEAE-Sephadex A50 chromatography of human plasma (M. E. Webster, personal communication). The elimination of differences in electrophoretic mobility in alkaline disc gels after neuraminidase treatment or after introduction of 8 M urea together with the small difference in sedimentation coefficient suggests a contribution of carbohydrate side-chain charge to the differing chromatographic properties (Spragg and Austen, 1974). These observations are further strengthened by the finding that the partial specific volumes of the two kininogens are dissimilar (Spragg and Austen, 1974). Such differences in carbohydrate content have been described for other glycoproteins (Schmid, 1968) and have recently been reported to account for the separation on DEAE-Sephadex A50 of two forms of bovine clotting factor X (Jackson, 1972). The observation that desialylated glycoproteins are more rapidly removed from the circulation than unmodified molecules on injection into rats (Morell *et al.*, 1971) raises the possibility that kininogen with less carbohydrate content may represent an early step in removal of this molecule from the circulation.

In contrast to the above, the use of an inhibitor of Hageman factor activation and mild purification conditions has resulted in the preparation of a single kininogen from human plasma having a molecular weight of 70,000 (Spragg and Austen, 1971) or 79,000 (Spragg *et al.*, 1973; Cochrane and Wuepper, 1971*a*; Wuepper and Cochrane, 1971) susceptible to both urinary and plasma kallikrein (Cochrane and Wuepper, 1971*a*; Spragg and Austen, 1971, 1974; Wuepper and Cochrane, 1971) and resistant to inactivation of the kinin moiety by carboxypeptidase B (Spragg and Austen, 1974). This last result is in accord with the finding that carboxypeptidase B releases a limited amount of arginine from purified bovine kininogen of molecular weight 70,000 and that the sensitive material increases as a result of purification (Suzuki *et al.*, 1973). A high degree of peptide homology has been found between bovine kininogens of molecular weight 70,000 and 50,000, leading to the proposal of a model of a single kininogen with the kinin moiety located internally which may undergo limited proteolysis to yield both altered high molecular weight kininogen and low molecular weight kininogen (Komiya *et al.*, 1972; Suzuki *et al.*, 1973). Thus a limited degree of proteolysis and variations in carbohydrate content may account for the apparent heterogeneity of the plasma proteins containing the nonapeptide bradykinin sequence.

3.7. Kininases

Two enzymes which inactivate bradykinin have been characterized and purified from human plasma or serum: kininase I, an arginine carboxypeptidase (Erdös and Sloane, 1962), and kininase II, which cleaves the carboxy-terminal phenylalanyl arginine dipeptide from bradykinin (Yang and Erdös, 1967). With regard to size, chromatographic properties, substrate specificity, and inhibition (Yang and Erdös, 1967), kininase I appears to be the same protein as the anaphylatoxin inactivator which has been purified from human serum by anion exchange chromatography, gel filtration, and electrophoresis (Bokisch and Müller-Eberhard, 1970). Anaphylatoxin inactivator, an α-globulin with a molecular weight of 325,000, cleaves the carboxy-terminal arginine from the human anaphylatoxins C3a and C5a and from bradykinin (Bokisch and Müller-Eberhard, 1970). Kininase II, which appears to have the same size as kininase I by Sephadex G200 gel filtration, has been separated from it by DEAE-Sephadex chromatography (Yang and Erdös, 1967). Kininase II appears to be identical to the carboxydipeptidase angiotensin I converting enzyme (Yang *et al.*, 1970, 1971; Engel *et al.*, 1972).

In addition to the kininases identified as active plasma enzymes, kinin-inactivating activities have also been observed in formed elements of the blood (Erdös and Yang, 1970) (Section 5).

4. METHODS OF ASSAY

4.1. Functional Assays

Hageman factor has been measured by its ability to correct the partial thromboplastin time of Hageman factor deficient plasma, activate prekallikrein, or hydrolyze N-α-acetylglycine lysine methyl ester (Kaplan and Austen, 1971; Cochrane and Wuepper, 1971b; Ulevitch and Letchford, 1973); kallikrein, by its ability to release bradykinin from kininogen or to cleave certain synthetic esters (Webster and Pierce, 1963; Colman et al., 1969; Wuepper and Cochrane, 1971); plasminogen activator, by its capacity to convert plasminogen to plasmin in the absence of streptokinase or urokinase (Kaplan and Austen, 1972); plasmin, by its caseinolytic, fibrinolytic, or esterolytic capacity (Robbins et al., 1965; Kaplan and Austen, 1972); kininogen, by its ability to serve as a substrate for kinin-generating enzymes (Diniz and Carvalho, 1963; Pierce and Webster, 1966); and bradykinin, by a variety of bioassays based on its pharmacological properties, in particular its ability to contract the guinea pig ileum or estrous rat uterus or to lower the blood pressure in isolated limb preparations (reviewed by Trautschold, 1970).

4.2. Immunological Methods for Measuring Certain Components of the Kinin-Forming System

Because of the ease with which the Hageman factor dependent systems are activated and the presence of inhibitors of the enzyme components of the activation pathways, as well as the presence of at least two kinin-destroying enzymes, functional assays have limitations; therefore, monospecific antibodies directed against several of the components of this system have been employed for the development of clinically useful immunoassays. Preparation of antibody against human Hageman factor (Cochrane et al., 1972c; Ratnoff, 1972), plasminogen (Robbins and Summaria, 1966), kininogen (Spragg et al., 1970a; Spragg and Austen, 1971), and bradykinin (reviewed by Spragg et al., 1970b) has been described. The last three have been incorporated in clinical immunoassays, namely, radial immunodiffusion assays for kininogen (Spragg et al., 1974; Wintroub et al., 1973) and plasminogen/plasmin (Magoon et al., 1974a,b) and radioimmunoassays for plasminogen/plasmin (Rabiner et al., 1968) and bradykinin (Goodfriend and Ball, 1969; Mashford and Roberts, 1972; Rinderknecht et al., 1967; Talamo et al., 1969; Wintroub et al., 1973).

4.2.1. Radial Immunoassay for Kininogen

The functional assay for kininogen in whole plasma requires heat and acid treatment to destroy the kinin-forming enzymes and their inhibitors (Diniz and Carvalho, 1963). The kininogen denatured by this procedure exhibits reduced reactivity with plasma kallikrein (Habermann, 1970), and therefore trypsin is used as the kinin-releasing enzyme. As previously described, the kininogen levels determined by the functional assay using trypsin are in good agreement with the protein levels obtained on radial immunodiffusion (Spragg *et al.*, 1974; Wintroub *et al.*, 1973). When blood was collected in disodium ethylenediamine tetraacetic acid and hexadimethrine bromide, an inhibitor of Hageman factor activation, the mean kininogen level found in a group of 50 normal volunteers was 675 ± 170 μg per milliliter of plasma (Wintroub *et al.*, 1973).

4.2.2. Radioimmunoassay for Bradykinin

The radioimmunoassay for bradykinin used in this laboratory incorporates antibody directed against bradykinin coupled to ovalbumin, the hapten [^{125}I] Tyr^8-bradykinin, and IRC50 chromatography of the trichloroacetic acid supernatant of freshly collected biological fluids prior to assay (Talamo *et al.*, 1969). In order to eliminate antigenic cross-reacting material from the bradykinin-containing mixture, a QAE-Sephadex chromatographic procedure is presently performed prior to the IRC50 step. With this modification, results indicate that the recovery of bradykinin added to plasma is 70–80% whether assayed by radioimmunoassay or bioassay (Wintroub *et al.*, 1973). The apparent plasma level of 5 ± 2 mμg/ml found in 19 normal individuals may reflect generation during harvesting and processing rather than the true endogenous bradykinin level.

4.2.3. Radial Immunoassay for Plasminogen and Plasmin

In contrast to earlier preparations of a plasminogen immunogen by isoelectric precipitation, chromatography, and gel filtration of human Cohn fraction III$_{2,3}$ (see Section 3.4) (Robbins and Summaria, 1966), the present assay is based on the use of an immunogen prepared from fresh nondenatured, nonprecipitated plasma by affinity chromatography (Deutsch and Mertz, 1970). Rabbits were immunized with plasminogen in complete Freund's adjuvant, and the antiserum collected was adsorbed with IgG-Sepharose to render it monospecific for plasminogen/plasmin. Such antiserum was incorporated in a radial immunodiffusion assay standardized on a weight and functional basis with highly purified plasminogen also prepared from fresh plasma without denaturation; in a series of 30 normal individuals, the plasma plasminogen/plasmin level was found to be 476 μg/ml (Magoon *et al.*, 1974a,b), a level considerably higher than that found in the radioimmunoassay (200 μg/ml, Rabiner *et al.*, 1968).

5. COMPONENTS OF THE KININ SYSTEM IN WHITE BLOOD CELLS

The conditions under which kinins are generated by leukocyte enzymes experimentally, the limited characterization of possible substrates for these enzymes, and the presence of kininases in the same cell types do not at present permit an understanding of an *in vivo* role for the white cell kinin-forming enzymes or their products. However, because of their possible participation in an inflammatory response mediated by plasma components, they are considered here.

5.1. Kinin-Forming Enzymes and Leukokinins

When whole cell lysates (Greenbaum and Yamafuji, 1966) and lysosomal (pellet) or extralysosomal (supernatant) cell fractions (Greenbaum and Kim, 1967) from rabbit peritoneal polymorphonuclear leukocyte (PMN) exudates were incubated for several hours at pH 3.5 with partially purified human kininogen prepared from outdated human whole blood, material was generated which contracted the guinea pig ileum. The destruction of this material by carboxypeptidase B and chymotrypsin (Greenbaum and Yamafuji, 1966; Greenbaum and Kim, 1967) led to its designation as "PMN-kinin." As studies were expanded to enzymes obtained from human lymphocytes (Engleman and Greenbaum, 1971) and rabbit alveolar and peritoneal macrophages (Greenbaum *et al.*, 1969), the more general term "leukokinin" was proposed (Chang *et al.*, 1972) for the biological activity generated.

The kinin-forming activity was found in lysosomal, extralysosomal, and nuclear debris fractions in the cell types examined and was shown to have a different inhibition profile from that of plasma kallikrein (Greenbaum *et al.*, 1969; Engleman and Greenbaum, 1971). When a PMN lysosomal fraction lacking the ability to destroy bradykinin was examined with regard to the pH optimum of its kinin-forming activity, it was apparent that the source and method of purifying the substrate were important, the enzyme having a pH optimum of about 4–5 with human kininogen and a pH optimum of 7–8 with highly purified bovine kininogen (Greenbaum and Kim, 1967). The nature of the kinins formed also appeared to depend on the source of enzyme and substrate employed (Greenbaum *et al.*, 1969). As determined by kinin generation and kininogen depletion, kinin-forming activity with both a neutral and an acidic pH optimum was identified when whole human granulocytes or an extralysosomal supernatant was incubated with whole plasma (Melmon and Cline, 1968). Although a role for Hageman factor was suggested since cells were inactive in Hageman factor deficient plasma, purified kininogen or heat-inactivated normal plasma was capable of providing a substrate for kinin-generating and kininogen-depleting activity (Melmon and Cline, 1968).

The leukokinin obtained from the incubation of extralysosomal PMN enzymes with human kininogen (leukokinin PMN) and the last of four fractions recovered from CM-cellulose chromatography of kinins obtained when a whole cell lysate of alveolar macrophages was used as an enzyme source (leukokinin M) were further purified and characterized. The former had a molecular weight of 2416, and the latter of 2826. The recovery of fewer than two phenylalanine residues in both peptides and the presence in leukokinin M of one of the two arginines in a sequence unlike that of bradykinin suggest that these peptides do not contain the bradykinin sequence (Chang *et al.*, 1972); their relative potency in eight bioassay systems is different from that of bradykinin (Freer *et al.*,

Although the substrate employed for the generation of leukokinins by Greenbaum and Kim (1967), Greenbaum *et al.* (1969), and Chang *et al.* (1972) has been purified plasma kininogen of human, rabbit, or bovine origin, these authors have recently stated that purified kininogens are not substrates for leukokinin-forming enzymes (Greenbaum and Nagasawa, 1971; Greenbaum *et al.*, 1972). Further examination of a substrate for these enzymes has been limited to whole plasma or ascites fluid (Greenbaum, 1972).

5.2. Kininases

Kinin-destroying activity of leukocytes (Schwab, 1962; Zachariae *et al.*, 1966) has been further identified in the extralysosomal fraction of rabbit PMN cells (Greenbaum and Kim, 1967) and alveolar macrophages (Greenbaum *et al.*, 1969) and shown to have an inhibition profile different from that of plasma kininases (Greenbaum *et al.*, 1969). Although these cell fractions destroy both leukokinins M and PMN (Greenbaum *et al.*, 1969; Chang *et al.*, 1972), the alkaline pH optimum (Greenbaum and Kim, 1967) and the inhibition profile have been determined using bradykinin rather than leukokinins and incubation periods of 30–60 min rather than the 16 h employed in leukokinin-generating experiments. Bradykinin-destroying activity has also been demonstrated in intact and disrupted human granulocytes; at pH 7.4 activity was largely in the nuclear debris and supernatant fractions, while at pH 5.5 increased kininase activity was observed in the pellet fraction (Melmon and Cline, 1968).

6. ROLE OF THE KININ-FORMING SYSTEM IN INFLAMMATION

In spite of the many recent advances in characterizing the components and interactions in the kinin-forming pathway, the exact role of this system in an *in vivo* inflammatory response has yet to be determined. Individuals who lack either Hageman factor or prekallikrein appear clinically normal (Ratnoff *et al.*, 1968; Hathaway *et al.*, 1965; Wuepper, 1972), and studies of models of inflammation are difficult to interpret because of the complexity of the kinin-forming system and its interactions with other plasma systems. The ease of artifactually activating this system and the rapidity with which bradykinin is destroyed in the circulation ($t_{1/2}$ = 20 s) further complicate such studies. Accumulated evidence would suggest a secondary role for the kinin-forming pathway, possibly dependent on the exposure of surfaces or activation of enzymes capable of converting Hageman factor to an active form (see Section 6.1). Subsequent conversion of the Hageman factor substrates to their active enzymatic forms could then lead to the generation of several biological activities capable of contributing to an inflammatory response either directly or by interaction with other systems (see Section 6.2).

6.1. Activation of Hageman Factor

Early studies of Hageman factor activation using nonbiological surfaces have been extended to such negatively charged surfaces as collagen (Niewiarowski *et al.*, 1965; Wilner *et al.*, 1968), articular cartilage (Moskowitz *et al.*, 1970), elastin (Niewiarowski *et al.*, 1965), renal vascular basement membrane (Cochrane *et al.*, 1972a), and the sodium urate crystals of gout and the pyrophosphate crystals of pseudogout (Kellermeyer and Breckenridge, 1965). Surface binding of Hageman factor has been demonstrated in studies employing elastin and collagen (Niewiarowski *et al.*, 1965) and vascular basement membrane (Cochrane *et al.*, 1972a). Fragmentation of Hageman factor, which leads to a more acidic isoelectric point (see Section 3.2), is associated with a loss of binding to negatively charged surfaces (Webster, 1972). The enzymes kallikrein, plasmin, and trypsin activate Hageman factor (Cochrane *et al.*, 1972a); PTA is also said to be an activator (Revak *et al.*, 1973; Cochrane *et al.*, 1973). A soluble lipopolysaccharide from *Escherichia coli* converts Hageman factor to the active form, the presence of phosphate groups being associated with activation (Cochrane *et al.*, 1973).

Following the original observation of Beraldo (1950) that kinin was released in active anaphylaxis in the dog, activation of the kinin-forming system has been examined in numerous models of experimental anaphylaxis (reviewed by Spragg *et al.*, 1970b; Wintroub *et al.*, 1973). *In vitro* activation of this system in whole serum with antigen–antibody aggregates (Davies and Lowe, 1962; Eisen and Smith, 1970; Epstein *et al.*, 1969; Movat and DiLorenzo, 1968; Movat *et al.*, 1968) and of purified human Hageman factor with a soluble immune complex (Kaplan *et al.*, 1971) has been reported. Antigen–antibody aggregates have been shown to be weak activators of rabbit precursor prokininogenase activator

(Tucker and Wuepper, 1969; Cochrane and Wuepper, 1971a), but the most recent investigations have failed to demonstrate immunological activation of purified Hageman factor from rabbit or man (Cochrane et al., 1972c). Although these last experiments examined a possible requirement for plasma or serum in activation of Hageman factor by preformed complexes, formation of complexes in the presence of plasma or serum as in earlier experiments may be required for binding of potential activating materials such as the collagen-like molecule C1q (Yonemasu et al., 1971).

6.2. Interaction with Other Plasma Systems

From the discussion above (see Section 2), it is apparent that the components of the kinin-forming pathway may interact in many ways with other plasma systems. The intrinsic coagulation pathway is initiated by Hageman factor, whose activation is amplified by PTA, kallikrein, and plasmin (see Section 6.1). The conversion of human fibrinogen to fibrin by thrombin generates a fibrinopeptide designated "β-peptide" (Osbahr et al., 1963) (human fibrinopeptide A of Blombäck et al., 1966) which enhances the bradykinin-induced contraction of smooth muscle preparations (Osbahr et al., 1964). Fibrinopeptide B has chemotactic activity (Kay et al., 1973). The Hageman factor dependent conversion of plasminogen to plasmin may result not only in fibrinolytic activity but also in the attendant formation of fibrinogen and fibrin degradation products with anticoagulant, permeability, or chemotactic activity (see Section 2.3). Plasmin-induced activation of the complement sequence results in the generation of numerous biological activities.

In addition to the generation of chemotactic activities via coagulation and fibrinolysis and through activation of the complement sequence, both kallikrein and plasminogen activator are themselves chemotactic. The possibility that bradykinin may release histamine from cellular stores has been examined using rat peritoneal mast cells (Johnson and Erdös, 1973) and is supported by the observation that antihistamines diminish the bradykinin-induced vascular permeability in the skin of several species (Becker et al., 1968).

The multiple points of action of the inhibitors of this system (see Section 2.6 and Table I) as well as their ability to inhibit certain enzymes in other plasma systems constitute another point of interaction. It is likely that still others remain to be elucidated.

7. REFERENCES

Amir, J., Ratnoff, O. D., and Pensky, J., 1972, Partial purification and some properties of a plasma inhibitor of activated plasma thromboplastin antecedent (factor XI), *J. Lab. Clin. Med.* **80:**786.

Barlow, G. H., Summaria, L., and Robbins, K. C., 1969, Molecular weight studies on human plasminogen and plasmin at the microgram level, *J. Biol. Chem.* 244:1138.

Barnhart, M. I., Sulisz, L., and Bluhm, G. B., 1971, Role for fibrinogen and its derivatives in acute inflammation, in: *Immunopathology of Inflammation* (B. K. Forscher and J. C. Houck, eds.), pp. 59–65, Excerpta Medica, Amsterdam.

Becker, E. L., Mota, I., and Wong, D., 1968, Inhibition by antihistamines of the vascular permeability increase induced by bradykinin, *Brit. J. Pharmacol.* 34:330.

Beraldo, W. T., 1950, Formation of bradykinin in anaphylactic and peptone shock, *Am. J. Physiol.* 163:283.

Blombäck, B., Blombäck, M., Edman, P., and Hessel, B., 1966, Human fibrinopeptides, isolation, characterization and structure, *Biochim. Biophys. Acta* 115:371.

Boissonnas, R. A., Guttman, S., Jaquenoud, P. A., Konzett, H., and Stürmer, E., 1960, Synthesis and biological activity of peptides related to bradykinin, *Experientia* 16:326.

Bokisch, V. A., and Müller-Eberhard, H. J., 1970, Anaphylatoxin inactivator of human plasma: Its isolation and characterization as a carboxypeptidase, *J. Clin. Invest.* 49:2427.

Burrowes, C. E., Movat, H. Z., and Soltay, M. J., 1971, The kinin system of human plasma. VI. The action of plasmin, *Proc. Soc. Exp. Biol. Med.* 138:959.

Chang, J., Freer, R., Stella, R., and Greenbaum, L. M., 1972, Studies on leukokinins. II. Studies on the formation, partial amino acid sequence and chemical properties of leukokinins M and PMN, *Biochem. Pharmacol.* 21:3095.

Cochrane, C. G., and Wuepper, K. D., 1971*a*, The kinin-forming system: Delineation and activation, in: *VIth International Symposium of Immunopathology* (P. A. Miescher, ed.), pp. 220–235, Benno-Schwabe, Basel.

Cochrane, C. G., and Wuepper, K. D., 1971*b*, The first component of the kinin-forming system in human and rabbit plasma: Its relationship to clotting factor XII (Hageman factor), *J. Exp. Med.* 134:986.

Cochrane, C. G., Revak, S. D., Aiken, B. S., and Wuepper, K. D., 1972*a*, The structural characteristics and activation of Hageman factor, in: *Inflammation: Mechanisms and Control* (I. H. Lepow and P. A. Ward, eds.), pp. 119–138, Academic Press, New York.

Cochrane, C. G., Sitzer, S. D., and Aiken, B. S., 1972*b*, Hageman factor, its structure and activation, *Fed. Proc.* 31:623 (abst.).

Cochrane, C. G., Wuepper, K. D., Aiken, B. S., Revak, S. D., and Spiegelberg, H. L., 1972*c*, The interaction of Hageman factor and immune complexes, *J. Clin. Invest.* 51:2736.

Cochrane, C. G., Revak, S. D., Wuepper, K. D., and Morrison, D., 1973, The structural characteristics of Hageman factor, in: *VIIth International Symposium of Immunopathology* (abst.).

Colman, R. W., Mattler, L., and Sherry, S., 1969, Studies on the prekallikrein (Kallikreinogen)–kallikrein enzyme system of human plasma. I. Isolation and purification of plasma kallikrein, *J. Clin. Invest.* 48:11.

Davies, G. E., and Lowe, J. S., 1962, Further studies on a permeability factor released from guinea pig serum by antigen–antibody precipitates: Relationship to serum complement, *Int. Arch. Allergy Appl. Immunol.* 20:235.

Deutsch, D. G., and Mertz, E. T., 1970, Plasminogen: Purification from human plasma by affinity chromatography, *Science* 170:1095.

Diniz, C. R., and Čarvalho, I. F., 1963, A micromethod for determination of bradykininogen under several conditions, *Ann. N.Y. Acad. Sci.* 104:77.

Eisen, V., and Smith, H. G., 1970, Plasma kinin formation by complexes of gamma globulin and serum proteins, *Brit. J. Exp. Pathol.* 51:328.

Elliott, D. F., Lewis, G. P., and Horton, E. W., 1960, The structure of bradykinin–A plasma kinin from ox blood, *Biochem. Biophys. Res. Commun.* 3:87.

Engel, S. L., Schaeffer, T. R., Gold, B. I., and Rubin, B., 1972, Inhibition of pressor effects of angiotensin I and augmentation of depressor effects of bradykinin by synthetic peptides, *Proc. Soc. Exp. Biol. Med.* **140**:240.

Engelman, E. G., and Greenbaum, L. M., 1971, Kinin-forming activity of human lymphocytes, *Biochem. Pharmacol.* **20**:922.

Epstein, W. V., Tan, M., and Melmon, K. L., 1969, Rheumatoid factor and kinin generation, *Ann. N.Y. Acad. Sci.* **168**:173.

Erdös, E. G., 1966, Hypotensive peptides: bradykinin, kallidin and eledoisin, *Advan. Pharmacol.* **4**:1–90.

Erdös, E. G. (ed.), 1970, *Handbook of Experimental Pharmacology*, Vol. XXV, Springer-Verlag, Berlin.

Erdös, E. G., and Sloane, E. M., 1962, An enzyme in human blood plasma that inactivates bradykinin and kallidins, *Biochem. Pharmacol.* **11**:585.

Erdös, E. G., and Yang, H. Y. T., 1970, Kininases, in: *Handbook of Experimental Pharmacology*, Vol. XXV (E. G. Erdös, ed.), pp. 289–323, Springer-Verlag, Berlin.

Forbes, C. B., Pensky, J., and Ratnoff, O. D., 1970, Inhibition of activated Hageman factor and activated plasma thromboplastin antecedent by purified CĪ inactivator, *J. Lab. Clin. Med.* **76**:809.

Freer, R., Chang, J., and Greenbaum, L. M., 1972, Studies on leukokinins. III. Pharmacological activities of leukokinins M and PMN, *Biochem. Pharmacol.* **21**:3107.

Fritz, H., Wunderer, G., Kummer, K., Heimburger, N., and Werle, E., 1972, a_1-Antitrypsin und CĪ Inaktivator: Progressiv-inhibitoren für Serumkallikreine von Mensch und Schwein, *Z. Physiol. Chem.* **353**:906.

Gigli, I., Ruddy, S., and Austen, K. F., 1968, The stoichiometric measurement of the serum inhibitor of the first component of complement by the inhibition of immune hemolysis, *J. Immunol.* **100**:1154.

Gigli, I., Mason, J. W., Colman, R. W., and Austen, K. F., 1970, Interaction of plasma kallikrein with the CĪ inhibitor, *J. Immunol.* **104**:574.

Goetzel, E. J., and Austen, K. F., 1974, Active site chemotactic factors and the regulation of the human neutrophil chemotactic response, in: *Chemotaxis: Its Biology and Biochemistry* (E. Sorkin, ed.), in press, Karger, Basel.

Goodfriend, T. L., and Ball, D. B., 1969, Radioimmunoassay of bradykinin: Chemical modification to enable use of radioactive iodine, *J. Lab. Clin. Med.* **73**:501.

Graham, R. C., Jr., Ebert, R. H., Ratnoff, O. D., and Moses, J. M., 1965, Pathogenesis of inflammation. II. *In vivo* observations of the inflammatory effects of activated Hageman factor and bradykinin, *J. Exp. Med.* **121**:807.

Greenbaum, L. M., 1972, Leukocyte kininogenases and leukokinins from normal and malignant cells, *Am. J. Pathol.* **68**:613.

Greenbaum, L. M., and Kim, K. S., 1967, The kinin-forming and kininase activities of rabbit polymorphonuclear leukocytes, *Brit. J. Pharmacol. Chemother.* **29**:238.

Greenbaum, L. M., and Nagasawa, S., 1971, Substrates other than bradykininogen which release kinins in the presence of white cell enzymes, *Pharmacologist* **13**:214 (abst.).

Greenbaum, L. M., and Yamafuji, K., 1966, The role of cathepsins in the inactivation of plasma kinins, in: *Hypotensive Peptides* (E. G. Erdös, N. Back, and F. Sicuteri, eds.), pp. 252–262, Springer-Verlag, Berlin.

Greenbaum, L. M., Freer, R., Chang, J., Semente, G., and Yamafuji, K., 1969, PMN-kinin and kinin metabolizing enzymes in normal and malignant leukocytes, *Brit. J. Pharmacol.* **36**:623.

Greenbaum, L. M., Semente, G. R., and Prakash, A., 1972, Studies on leukokininogen in human plasma, *Fed. Proc.* **31**:534 (abst.).

Habal, R. M., and Movat, H. Z., 1972, Kininogens of human plasma, *Res. Commun. Chem. Pathol. Pharmacol.* **4**:477.

Habermann, E., 1970, Kininogens, in: *Handbook of Experimental Pharmacology*, Vol. XXV (E. G. Erdös, ed.), pp. 250–288, Springer-Verlag, Berlin.

Harpel, P. C., 1970, Human plasma alpha 2-macroglobulin, an inhibitor of plasma kallikrein, *J. Exp. Med.* **132**:329.

Harpel, P. C., 1971, Separation of plasma thromboplastin antecedent from kallikrein by the plasma α_2-macroglobulin, kallikrein inhibitor, *J. Clin. Invest.* **50**:2084.

Hathaway, W. E., Belhasen, L. P., and Hathaway, H. S., 1965, Evidence for a new plasma thromboplastin factor. I. Case report, coagulation studies and physicochemical properties, *Blood* **26**:521.

Jackson, C. B., 1972, Characterization of two glycoprotein variants of bovine factor X and demonstration that the factor X zymogen contains two polypeptide chains, *Biochemistry* **11**:4873.

Jacobsen, S., 1966, Substrates for plasma kinin-forming enzymes in human, dog, and rabbit plasmas, *Brit. J. Pharmacol.* **26**:403.

Jacobsen, S., and Kriz, M., 1967, Some data on two purified kininogens from human plasma, *Brit. J. Pharmacol. Chemother.* **29**:25.

Johnson, A. R., and Erdös, E. G., 1973, Release of histamine from mast cells by vasoactive peptides, *Proc. Soc. Exp. Biol. Med.* **142**:1252.

Johnston, A. R., Cochrane, C. G., and Revak, S. D., 1974, The relationship between PF/dil and activated human Hageman factor, *J. Immunol.* **113**:103.

Kagan, L. J., 1964, Some biochemical and physical properties of the human permeability globulins, *Brit. J. Exp. Pathol.* **45**:604.

Kagan, L. J., Leddy, J. P., and Becker, E. L., 1963, The presence of two permeability globulins in human serum, *J. Clin. Invest.* **42**:1353.

Kaplan, A. P., and Austen, K. F., 1970, A prealbumin activator of prekallikrein, *J. Immunol.* **105**:802.

Kaplan, A. P., and Austen, K. F., 1971, A prealbumin activator of prekallikrein. II. Derivation of activators of prekallikrein from active Hageman factor by digestion with plasmin, *J. Exp. Med.* **133**:696.

Kaplan, A. P., and Austen, K. F., 1972, The fibrinolytic pathway of human plasma: Isolation and characterization of the plasminogen proactivator, *J. Exp. Med.* **136**:1378.

Kaplan, A. P., Spragg, J., and Austen, K. F., 1971, The bradykinin-forming system of man, in: *Second International Symposium on the Biochemistry of the Acute Allergic Reactions* (K. F. Austen and E. L. Becker, eds.), pp. 279–298, Blackwell, Oxford.

Kaplan, A. P., Kay, A. B., and Austen, K. F., 1972, A prealbumin activator of prekallikrein. III. Appearance of chemotactic activity for human neutrophils by the conversion of human prekallikrein to kallikrein, *J. Exp. Med.* **135**:81.

Kaplan, A. P., Goetzl, E. J., and Austen, K. F., 1973, The fibrinolytic pathway of human plasma. II. The generation of chemotactic activity by activation of plasminogen proactivator, *J. Clin. Invest.* **52**:2591.

Kay, A. B., Pepper, D. S., and Ewart, M. R., 1973, Generation of chemotactic activity for leukocytes by the action of thrombin on human fibrinogen, *Nature New Biol.* **243**:56.

Kellermeyer, R. W., and Breckenridge, R. T., 1965, The inflammatory process in acute gouty arthritis. I. Activation of Hageman factor by sodium urate crystals, *J. Lab. Clin. Med.* **65**:307.

Komiya, M., Kata, H., and Suzuki, T., 1972, Homology between bovine high molecular weight and low molecular weight kininogens, *Biochem. Biophys. Res. Commun.* **49**:1438.

Lewis, G. P., 1958, Formation of plasma kinins by plasmin, *J. Physiol. (Lond.)* 140:285.

MacKay, M. W., Miles, A. A., Schachter, M., and Wilhelm, D. L., 1953, Susceptibility of the guinea pig to pharmacological factors from its own serum, *Nature (Lond.)* 172:714.

Magoon, E. H., Spragg, J., and Austen, K. J., 1974a, Human Hageman factor dependent pathways, in *Advances in Biosciences, vol. 12* (G. Raspé, ed.), pp. 225–236, Pergamon Press Vieweg, Braunschweig.

Magoon, E. H., Austen, K. F., and Spragg, J., 1974b, Immunoelectrophoretic analysis and radial immunodiffusion using plasminogen purified from fresh human plasma, *Clin. Exp. Immunol.* 17:345.

Marder, V. J., and Shulman, N. R., 1969, High molecular weight derivatives of human fibrinogen produced by plasmin. II. Mechanism of their anticoagulant activity, *J. Biol. Chem.* 244:2120.

Mashford, M. L., and Roberts, M. L., 1972, Determination of blood kinin levels by radioimmunoassay, *Biochem. Pharmacol.* 21:2727.

Mason, B., and Miles, A. A., 1962, Globulin permeability factors without kininogenase activity, *Nature (Lond.)* 196:587.

McConnell, D. J., 1972, Inhibitors of kallikrein in human plasma, *J. Clin. Invest.* 51:1611.

Melmon, K. L., and Cline, M. J., 1968, The interaction of leukocytes and the kinin system, *Biochem. Pharmacol. Suppl.:* 271.

Merrifield, R. B., 1964, Solid phase peptide synthesis. III. An improved synthesis of bradykinin, *Biochemistry* 3:1385.

Morell, A. G., Gregoriadis, G., Scheinberg, I. H., Hickman, J., and Ashwell, G., 1971, The role of sialic acid in determining the survival of glycoproteins in the circulation, *J. Biol. Chem.* 246:1461.

Moskowitz, R. W., Schwartz, H. J., Michel, B., Ratnoff, O. D., and Astrup, T., 1970, Generation of kinin-like agents by chondroitin sulfate, heparin, chitin sulfate, and human articular cartilage: Possible pathophysiologic implications, *J. Lab. Clin. Med.* 76:790.

Movat, H. Z., and DiLorenzo, N. L., 1968, Activation of the plasma kinin system by antigen–antibody aggregates. I. Generation of permeability factor in guinea pig serum, *Lab. Invest.* 19:187.

Movat, H. Z., DiLorenzo, N. L., and Treloar, M. D., 1968, Activation of the plasma kinin system by antigen–antibody aggregates. II. Isolation of permeability-enhancing and kinin releasing fractions from activated guinea pig serum, *Lab. Invest.* 19:201.

Movat, H. Z., Poon, M. C., and Takeuchi, Y., 1971, The kinin system of human plasma. I. Isolation of a low molecular weight activator of prekallikrein, *Int. Arch. Allergy Appl. Immunol.* 40:89.

Niewiarowski, S., Bankowski, E., and Rogowicka, I., 1965, Studies in the adsorption and activation of the Hageman factor (factor XII) by collagen and elastin, *Thromb. Diath. Haemorrh.* 14:387.

Norman, P. S., and Hill, B. M., 1958, Studies of the plasma system. III. Physical properties of the two plasmin inhibitors in plasma, *J. Exp. Med.* 108:639.

Ogston, D., Ogston, C. M., Ratnoff, O. D., and Forbes, C. D., 1969, Studies on a complex mechanism for the activation of plasminogen by kaolin and by chloroform: The participation of Hageman factor and additional cofactors, *J. Clin. Invest.* 48:1786.

Ogston, D., Bennett, N. B., Ogston, C. M., and Ratnoff, O. D., 1971, The assay of a plasma component necessary for the generation of a plasminogen activator in the presence of Hageman factor (Hageman factor co-factor), *Brit. J. Haematol.* 20:209.

Osbahr, A. J., Jr., Gladner, J. A., and Laki, K., 1963, The action of human thrombin on human fibrinogen, *Biochem. Biophys. Res. Commun.* 13:462.

Osbahr, A. J., Gladner, J. A., and Laki, K., 1964, Studies on the physiological activity of the peptide released during the fibrinogen–fibrin conversion, *Biochim. Biophys. Acta* 86:535.

Özge-Anwar, H., Ayse, H., Movat, H. Z., and Scott, J. G., 1972, The kinin system of human plasma. IV. The interrelationship between the contact phase of blood coagulation and the plasma kinin system in man, *Thromb. Diath. Haemorrh.* 27:141.

Pierce, J. V., 1968, Structural features of plasma kinins and kininogens, *Fed. Proc.* 27:52.

Pierce, J. V., and Webster, M. E., 1966, The purification and some properties of two different kallidinogens from human plasma, in: *Hypotensive Peptides* (E. G. Erdös, N. Back, and F. Sicuteri, eds.), pp. 130–138, Springer-Verlag, New York.

Rabiner, S. F., Goldfine, I. D., Hart, A., Summaria, L., and Robbins, K. C., 1968, Radioimmunoassay of human plasminogen and plasmin, *J. Lab. Clin. Med.* 74:216.

Ratnoff, O. D., 1965, Increased vascular permeability induced by human plasmin, *J. Exp. Med.* 122:905.

Ratnoff, O. D., 1972, Studies on the product of the reaction between activated Hageman factor (factor XII) and plasma thromboplastin antecedent (factor XI), *J. Lab. Clin. Med.* 80:704.

Ratnoff, O. D., and Miles, A. A., 1964, The induction of permeability-increasing activity in human plasma by activated Hageman factor, *Brit. J. Exp. Pathol.* 45:328.

Ratnoff, O. D., and Naff, G. B., 1967, The conversion of $C'1s$ to $C'1$ esterase by plasmin and trypsin, *J. Exp. Med.* 125:337.

Ratnoff, O. D., Davie, E. W., and Mallett, D. L., 1961, Studies on the action of Hageman factor: Evidence that activated Hageman factor in turn activates plasma thromboplastin antecedent, *J. Clin. Invest.* 40:803.

Ratnoff, O. D., Busse, R. J., Jr., and Sheon, R. P., 1968, The demise of John Hageman, *New Engl. J. Med.* 279:760.

Ratnoff, O. D., Pensky, J., Ogston, D., and Naff, G. B., 1969, The inhibition of plasmin, plasma kallikrein, plasma permeability factor, and the C1r subcomponent of the first component of complement by serum $C'1$ esterase inhibitor, *J. Exp. Med.* 129:315.

Revak, S. D., Cochrane, C. G., and Johnston, A. R., 1973, Structure of Hageman factor in its native and activated forms, *Fed. Proc.* 32:845 (abst.).

Righetti, P. G., and Drysdale, J. W., 1971, Isoelectric focusing in polyacrylamide gels, *Biochim. Biophys. Acta* 236:17.

Rinderknecht, H., Haverback, B. J., and Aladjem, F., 1967, Radioimmunoassay of bradykinin, *Nature (Lond.)* 213:1130.

Robbins, K. C., and Summaria, L., 1966, An immunochemical study of human plasminogen and plasmin, *Immunochemistry* 3:29.

Robbins, K. C., Summaria, L., Elwyn, D., and Barlow, G. H., 1965, Further studies on the purification and characterization of human plasminogen and plasmin, *J. Biol. Chem.* 240:541.

Rocha e Silva, M., 1970, *Kinin Hormones, with Special References to Bradykinin and Related Kinins*, Charles C Thomas, Springfield, Ill.

Schmid, K., 1968, Isolation, characterization and polymorphism of glycoproteins, in: *Biochemistry of Glycoproteins and Related Substances*, Part II: *Cystic Fibrosis* (E. Rossi and E. Stoll, eds.), pp. 4–58, Karger, Basel.

Schreiber, A. D., Kaplan, A. P., and Austen, K. F., 1973a, Inhibition by C1INH of Hageman factor fragment activation of coagulation, fibrinolysis, and kinin-generation, *J. Clin. Invest.* 52:1402.

Schreiber, A. D., Kaplan, A. P., and Austen, K. F., 1973b, Plasma inhibitors of the components of the fibrinolytic pathway in man, *J. Clin. Invest.* 52:1394.

Schwab, J., 1962, Kininases in leukocytes and other tissues, *Nature (Lond.)* 195:345.

Seidel, H., Stücker, H. U., and Vogt, W., 1969, The role of plasmin for kinin-formation in human plasma, *Naunyn-Schmiedebergs Arch. Pharmakol.* **264**:305 (abst.).

Seidel, G., Stücker, H. U., and Vogt, W., 1971, Significance of direct and indirect kinin formation by plasmin in human plasma, *Biochem. Pharmacol.* **20**:1859.

Soltay, M. J., Movat, H. Z., and Özge-Anwar, A. H., 1971, The kinin system of human plasma. V. The probable derivation of prekallikrein activator from activated Hageman factor, *Proc. Soc. Exp. Biol. Med.* **138**:952.

Spragg, J., and Austen, K. F., 1971, The preparation of human kininogen. II. Further characterization of purified human kininogen, *J. Immunol.* **107**:1512.

Spragg, J., and Austen, K. F., 1974, The preparation of human kininogen. III. Enzymatic digestion and modification, *Biochem. Pharmacol.* **23**:781.

Spragg, J., Haber, E., and Austen, K. F., 1970*a*, The preparation of human kininogen and the elicitation of antibody for use in a radial immunodiffusion assay, *J. Immunol.* **104**:1348.

Spragg, J., Talamo, R. C., and Austen, K. F., 1970*b*, Immunochemistry of bradykinin and immunologic activation of the kinin system, in: *Handbook of Experimental Pharmacology*, Vol. XXV (E. G. Erdös, ed.), Springer-Verlag, Berlin.

Spragg, J., Kaplan, A. P., and Austen, K. F., 1973, The use of isoelectric focusing to study components of the human plasma kinin-forming system, *Ann. N.Y. Acad. Sci.* **209**:372.

Spragg, J., Talamo, R. C., Wintroub, B. U., Haber, E., and Austen, K. F., 1974, Immunoassay of bradykinin and kininogen, in: *Methods in Immunology and Immunochemistry*, Vol. V (C. A. Williams and M. W. Chase, eds.), in press, Academic Press, New York.

Stecher, V. J., and Sorkin, E., 1972, The chemotactic activity of fibrin lysis products, *Int. Arch. Allergy* **43**:879.

Stewart, P. B., and Bliss, J. Q., 1957, The permeability-increasing factor in diluted human plasma, *Brit. J. Exp. Pathol.* **38**:462.

Suzuki, T., Kato, H., and Komiya, M., 1973, Biochemical properties of kininogens in plasma, in: *Proceedings of the Vth International Congress of Pharmacology*, pp. 296–306, Karger, Basel.

Talamo, R. C., Spragg, J., Haber, E., and Austen, K. F., 1969, Radioimmunoassay for bradykinin with an iodinated bradykinin analog and dextran coated charcoal, in: *Cellular and Humoral Mechanisms in Anaphylaxis and Allergy* (H. Z. Movat, ed.), pp. 226–232, Karger, Basel.

Trautschold, I., 1970, Assay methods in the kinin system, in: *Handbook of Experimental Pharmacology*, Vol. XXV (E. G. Erdös, ed.), pp. 52–81, Springer-Verlag, Berlin.

Treloar, M. P., and Movat, H. Z., 1970, Isolation of two small molecular weight activators of the plasma kinin-system in the guinea pig, *Fed. Proc.* **29**:576 (abst.).

Tucker, E. S., III, and Wuepper, K. D., 1969, Contact factor (CF) activation of rabbit kininogenase, *Fed. Proc.* **28**:363 (abst.).

Ulevitch, R. J., and Letchford, D. J., 1973, A direct enzymatic assay of Hageman factor activity, *Fed. Proc.* **32**:845 (abst.).

Vogt, W., 1964, Kinin formation by plasmin, an indirect process mediated by activation of kallikrein, *J. Physiol (Lond.)* **170**:153.

Ward, P. A., 1967, A plasmin-split fragment of C'3 as a new chemotactic factor, *J. Exp. Med.* **126**:189.

Webster, M., 1969, The kinin system—A review, in: *Cellular and Humoral Mechanisms in Anaphylaxis and Allergy* (H. Z. Movat, ed.), pp. 207–214, Karger, Basel.

Webster, M. E., 1972, The interaction of Hageman factor, prekallikrein activator and plasmin, in: *Proceedings of the Vth International Congress of Pharmacology*, p. 248 (abst.), Karger, Basel.

Webster, M. E., and Pierce, J. V., 1963, The nature of the kallidins released from human plasma by kallikreins and other enzymes, *Ann. N.Y. Acad. Sci.* **104**:91.

Weiss, A. S., Gallin, J. I., and Kaplan, A. P., 1973, Fletcher factor deficiency: Abnormalities of coagulation, fibrinolysis, chemotactic activity, and kinin generation attributable to absence of prekallikrein, *Fed. Proc.* 32:845 (abst.).

Weiss, A. S., Gallin, J. I., and Kaplan, A. P., 1974, Fletcher factor deficiency: a diminished rate of Hageman factor activation caused by absence of prekallikrein with abnormalities of coagulation, fibrinolysis, chemotactic activity and kinin generation, *J. Clin. Invest.* 53:622.

Wilner, G. D., Nossel, H. L., and LeRoy, E. C., 1968, Activation of Hageman factor by collagen, *J. Clin. Invest.* 47:2608.

Wintroub, B. U., Spragg, J., Stechschulte, D. J., and Austen, K. F., 1973, Characterization of and immunoassays for components of the kinin-generating system in: *Control Mechanisms in Reagin-Mediated Hypersensitivity* (L. Goodfriend, A. Sehon, and R. P. Orange, eds.), pp. 495–512, Marcel Dekker, New York.

Wuepper, K. D., 1972, Biochemistry and biology of components of the plasma kinin-forming system, in: *Inflammation: Mechanisms and Control* (I. H. Lepow and P. A. Ward, eds.), pp. 93–117, Academic Press, New York.

Wuepper, K. D., and Cochrane, C. G., 1971, Isolation and mechanism of activation of components of the plasma kinin-forming system, in: *Second International Symposium on the Biochemistry of the Acute Allergic Reactions* (K. F. Austen and E. L. Becker, eds.), pp. 299–320, Blackwell, Oxford.

Wuepper, K. D., and Cochrane, C. G., 1972, Plasma prekallikrein: Isolation, characterization, and mechanism of activation, *J. Exp. Med.* 135:1.

Wuepper, K. D., Tucker, E., III, and Cochrane, C. G., 1970, Plasma kinin system: Proenzyme components, *J. Immunol.* 105:1307.

Yang, H. Y. T., and Erdös, E. G., 1967, Second kininase in human blood plasma, *Nature (Lond.)* 215:1402.

Yang, H. Y. T., Erdös, E. G., and Levin, Y., 1970, A dipeptidyl carboxypeptidase that converts angiotensin I and inactivates bradykinin, *Biochim. Biophys. Acta* 214:374.

Yang, H. Y. T., Erdös, E. G., and Levin, Y., 1971, Characterization of a dipeptide hydrolase (kininase II: angiotensin I converting enzyme), *J. Pharmacol. Exp. Ther.* 177:291.

Yonemasu, K., Stroud, R. M., Niedermeier, W., and Butler, W. T., 1971, Chemical studies on C1q: a modulation of immunoglobulin biology, *Biochim. Biophys. Res. Commun.* 43:1388.

Zachariae, H., Malmquist, J., and Oates, J. A., 1966, Kininase in human polymorphonuclear leukocytes, *Life Sci.* 5:2347.

THE COMPLEMENT   4
AND PROPERDIN SYSTEMS

Shaun Ruddy

1. INTRODUCTION

From the original meaning of "complement" as the heat-labile substance present in serum and required for the killing of certain bacteria, the term "complement system" has evolved to denote a special group of normal serum proteins which interact sequentially to effect a variety of inflammatory events, including bacterial lysis. The term "properdin" was originally used to signify that substance in normal human serum which is required for zymosan to destroy the third component of complement, but has now come to designate a single protein among the four or five required for the zymosan-induced reaction. "Properdin system" is used to denote the entire sequence of serum proteins which participate in this reaction.

The application of techniques with high resolving power for such complex mixtures of proteins as human or guinea pig serum has permitted the isolation and partial chemical characterization of most of the constituents of the complement and properdin systems (Müller-Eberhard, 1968; Nelson *et al.*, 1966). The availability of purified reagents has permitted the definition, in molecular terms,

Dr. Ruddy is supported by an NIH Career Development Award (AM-70233).

SHAUN RUDDY Department of Medicine, Medical College of Virginia, Virginia Commonwealth University, Richmond, Virginia.

of the mechanisms of interaction of these proteins and the identification of multiple biological activities which attend complement and properdin activation (Ruddy *et al.*, 1972*a*). Products elaborated during these reactions mediate changes in vascular permeability, attract polymorphonuclear and mononuclear leukocytes, influence the release of lysosomal enzymes, bind to B-lymphocytes, enhance phagocytosis by promoting the adherence of complement-coated complexes to formed elements in the blood, and damage cell membranes to induce osmotic lysis and cell death. After a brief consideration of the nomenclature of the complement and properdin systems, each of these areas—chemistry, reaction mechanisms, and biological effects—will be considered in detail.

2. NOMENCLATURE

The names and commonly used synonyms of the complement and properdin system proteins are given in Table I. Ingredients of the complement system are known as "components," and by universal agreement (Austen *et al.*, 1968) they are symbolized by a capital "C" and a number designating the component, e.g., C1, C4, C2, C3. In the fluid phase, the activated state of the component is symbolized by a bar over the number, e.g., $\overline{C1}$, $\overline{C42}$; when bound to a particle such as a sheep erythrocyte (E) coated with rabbit antibody (A), components are assumed to be in their activated state and the bars are omitted, e.g., EAC1, EAC14. The molecular subunits of the macromolecular aggregate C1 are labeled C1q, C1r, and C1s (Lepow *et al.*, 1963). Cleavage fragments of components are suffixed with a,b,c,d,e.g., C3a, C3b (Bokisch *et al.*, 1969). The older names for components or fragments, based on their appearance in immunoelectrophoresis, e.g., β1C, β1E, β1F, β1A, are no longer accepted nomenclature.

Since the sequence and mechanisms of action of the factors of the properdin system are currently the subject of active investigation in a number of laboratories, there is no agreement about their nomenclature. "Properdin," the term initially (Pillemer *et al.*, 1954) used to signify the activity of all of the factors which have subsequently been described as required for the zymosan-induced inactivation of C3 in whole serum, is now used in a restricted sense to denote a single protein which is central to the zymosan reaction and has been obtained in a homogeneous form (Pensky *et al.*, 1968). Factor B, a heat-labile β-pseudo-globulin also required for the zymosan reaction (Blum *et al.*, 1959), is identical to the C3 proactivator (C3PA) (Götze and Müller-Eberhard, 1971) and glycine-rich β-glycoprotein (GBG) (Alper *et al.*, 1973). Factor D, a low molecular weight protein isolated during studies of the cobra venom factor (CoVF) induced destruction of C3 in serum (Hunsicker *et al.*, 1973), is the same as C3 proactivator convertase (C3PAase), (Müller-Eberhard and Götze, 1972, or GBGase

Table I. Physicochemical Characteristics of Proteins of the Complement and Properdin Systems

Name[a]	Molecular weight	Electro-phoretic mobility	Approximate Serum concentration (μg/ml)	Major fragments
Complement-system				
C1q	400,000	γ_2	190	
C1r	168,000	β		
C1s	90,000	β	120	
C4 (β_1E)	240,000	β_1	430	C4a, C4b
C2	117,000	β_2	30	C2a, C2b
C3 (β_1C)	185,000	β_1	1300	C3a, C3b, C3c (β_1A), C3d (α_2D)
C5(β_1F)	185,000	β_1	75	C5a, C5b
C6	125,000	β_2	60	
C7	120,000	β_2	60	
C8	150,000	γ_1	10	
C9	79,000	α	180	
Properdin system				
Properdin	186,000	γ_2	15	
Factor D (C3PAase, GBGase)	25,000	α_2	Trace	
Factor B (C3PA, GBG)	100,000	β_2	225	α-Fragment, GAG, γ-fragment, GGG
Control proteins				
C$\overline{1}$ inhibitor (E1)	90,000	α_2	180	
C3b inactivator (KAF)	100,000	β_2	25	
Anaphylatoxin inactivator	310,000	α		

[a]Synonyms are given in parentheses.

(Rosen and Alper, 1972). Factor A, the hydrazine-sensitive factor described in early studies of the properdin system, has been shown to be identical to native C3 (Müller-Eberhard and Götze, 1972), and factor C, found during studies of the CoVF-induced destruction of C3, appears to be the control protein, C3b inactivator (Ruddy *et al.*, 1973).

3. CHEMISTRY

The approximate molecular weights and electrophoretic mobilities of constituents of the complement and properdin systems are given in Table I. All are proteins, their concentrations ranging from a few micrograms per milliliter of human serum, as for factor D, C6, or C8, up to more than a milligram in the case of C3. Almost all have been tested and without exception found to be glycoproteins, with carbohydrate contents ranging from a few percent up to as high as 28% for C1 inhibitor (Pensky and Schwick, 1969). Most have molecular weights in the range of 100,000–200,000 and most have β-mobilities on electrophoresis, the last two features accounting, in part, for the difficulty with which these proteins are separated from each other. In addition to such general similarities, there appear to be definite homologies in the structures of certain of the components. For example, C3 and C5 have molecular weights, isoelectric points, and behavior on most ion exchange media which are extremely similar. On reduction and alkylation, both C3 and C5 consist of two subunits of approximately 115,000 and 75,000 mol wt, and the proteolytic cleavage of these components by trypsin and $C\overline{42}$ or $C\overline{423}$ appears to occur at a single peptide bond containing a basic amino acid. Both the C5a and C3a fragments liberated by these cleavage reactions have anaphylatoxic and chemotactic activity, albeit in varying amounts. From these similarities (Nilsson and Mapes, 1973), it seems likely that homologies may exist between the primary amino acid sequences of these two components. Another example of such chemical and functional similarity exists for C2, the protein which bears the active site for the classic C3 convertase, and factor B, which has an analogous position in a properdin system C3 convertase. Both are soluble at relatively high salt concentration, 2.2 M $(NH_4)_2SO_4$, and behave nearly identically on DEAE and CM-cellulose chromatography. The molecular weights of C2 and factor B are 120,000 and 100,000, respectively, and during activation fragments of 40,000 and 35,000 mol wt, respectively, are cleaved from the parent molecules, with the major portions of each protein participating in a Mg^+-dependent complex which has trypsin-like proteolytic activity.

3.1. Complement System

The activity of C1 resides in a multimolecular complex, approximately 1 million mol wt, whose integrity depends on the presence of Ca^{2+}. Chelation of this ion yields three proteins, C1q, C1r, and C1s, although the precise molar ratio of these subcomponents in the intact C1 molecule is as yet unclear. The C1q subunit, which contains the binding site of C1 for immunoglobulins, is both heat and acid labile, but is obtainable in high yield and purity by selective isoelectric precipitation (Yonemasu and Stroud, 1971) or by affinity chromatography on IgG-coated matrices (Bing, 1971). The C1q molecule appears to be unique among serum proteins in its content of hydroxylated amino acids and repeating glycines, which together with a characteristic disaccharide residue makes the C1q molecule extraordinarily similar to the structural protein, collagen. Intact C1q appears to contain two kinds of noncovalently linked subunits, six of 60,000 mol wt and two of 42,000 (Yonemasu and Stroud, 1972). Binding studies have shown that the valence of C1q for immunoglobulins is either 5 or 6, and electron microscopic studies have shown that the molecule consists of six terminal structures linked by radial connecting strands to a central core, which appears to have two smaller components. The terminal structures probably correspond to the 60,000 mol wt subunits and contain the binding sites for immunoglobulins; the two 42,000 mol wt fragments may form the central core. The collagen-like portions of the molecule, with the repeating glycines and the α-helical structure, may correspond to the connecting strands.

Although the mobility of C1s is listed as β, following activation to C1$\bar{s}$ a distinct anodal shift in mobility is apparent. This activation step, which can be catalyzed by trypsin, plasmin, or during complement activation by C1$\bar{r}$ (Valet and Cooper, 1973), appears to be associated with hydrolysis of a single peptide bond. Reduction and alkylation of native C1s yields a single chain, but the activated molecule contains two chains, one of 36,000 and the other of 77,000 mol wt. The active site of C1$\bar{s}$, as determined by binding of labeled diisopropyl fluorophosphate, appears to reside on the light chain (Sakai and Stroud, 1973). A very similar set of circumstances attends the activation of the serum protein plasminogen to the fibrinolytic enzyme plasmin: the parent molecule consists of a single chain, and activation to plasmin involves the cleavage of a single peptide bond, as revealed by the yield of two chains following reduction and alkylation of the active enzyme (Robbins *et al.*, 1967). Just as in the case of C1$\bar{s}$, the active site of plasmin appears to be on the light chain.

C4 and C2 are relatively difficult to isolate in quantity, so that although both have been purified to homogeneity and antibody directed against them has been prepared, little information is available about their subunit structure or amino acid sequence. Using the technique of antigen–antibody crossed electrophoresis, an inherited electrophoretic polymorphism of C4 has been demonstrated, although the mechanism of the genetic control is as yet incompletely understood (Rosenfeld *et al.*, 1969). The number of sulfhydryl groups in C2 has been titrated and found to be seven (Polley and Müller-Eberhard, 1969). Formation of one or more disulfide bridges among these SH groups is thought to be responsible for the tenfold increase in activity and resistance to temperature-dependent decay exhibited by C$\overline{42}$ formed from human C2 which has been lightly oxidized by treatment with iodine.

C3 was the first of the complement proteins to be purified (Müller-Eberhard, 1961), and this, together with the ready availability of antibody to this component, obtained simply by lightly immunizing animals with zymosan which has been incubated in human serum, accounts for the prevalence of C3 measurements in clinical medicine and the large number of immunofluorescence studies which have been performed with this component. On agarose gel electrophoresis of whole human serum, C3 is visible as a distinct band, and differences in the mobility of this band have been used to delineate an extensive genetic polymorphism of this component. Over 13 alleles have been described, and in any given individual two of these are inherited as autosomal codominants (Alper and Propp, 1968). The variations in subunit structure, amino acid sequence, or possibly carbohydrate residues which account for the observed differences in electrophoretic mobility have not been described. C5, which appears to be homologous to C3 in subunit structure and in functional behavior, does not appear to have a similar polymorphism.

C6 and C7 were the last two components (Inoue and Nelson, 1965, 1966) of the classic complement system to be identified as distinct entities, and only within the past year has the latter of these succumbed to attempts at purification (Arroyave and Müller-Eberhard, 1973). Antibody to human C6 has been prepared, but antibody to rabbit C6, which reacts with human C6, is more readily obtainable, since it can be produced simply by immunizing C6-deficient rabbits with normal rabbit serum; anti-C7 has also been reported. C8 is difficult to separate from IgG because of its similarity in net charge to these immunoglobulins, and treatment of highly purified fractions with anti-IgG immunoadsorbants is necessary to obtain a homogeneous preparation. By contrast, the major contaminant of C9 is often albumin, since this protein travels with C9 during the gel filtration step, which is useful for separating C9 from most of the other serum proteins and complement components; however, chromatography on cation exchange resins readily separates C9 from albumin.

3.2. Properdin System

Properdin itself, which was the first of the factors to be purified to homogeneity, appears to consist of four subunits of 45,000 mol wt (Minta and Lepow, 1973). Most purification procedures begin with a zymosan absorption step, in which the properdin contained in large volumes of serum is adsorbed to zymosan, the particles are washed, and the properdin is eluted in a small, highly enriched fraction. This appears to result in activation of the properdin, as assessed by its ability to induce C3 cleavage when introduced into whole serum, and thus far the purification of precursor properdin, which is distinguishable by a slight difference in mobility on immunoelectrophoresis (McClean and Michael,

1973) and by its failure to activate C3 in whole serum, has not been reported. Factor B, the heat-labile β-pseudoglobulin required for the zymosan-induced inactivation of C3 in whole serum, was purified independently and simultaneously as C3 proactivator (Götze and Müller-Eberhard, 1971) and as glycine-rich β-glycoprotein (Boenisch and Alper, 1970). Electrophoretic studies of GBG have demonstrated genetic polymorphism of this protein and are consistent with a tetrameric structure, assembled randomly from pools of two electrophoretically dissimilar subunits. Postulation of an additional subunit common to all GBG molecules was required to explain the observed heterogeneity of the cleavage products of this protein which appear following its activation (Alper et al., 1972a).

Factor D is a 25,000 mol wt protein which appears to be present in plasma partly in its activated form (Hunsicker et al., 1973) and partly in a trypsin-activatable precursor form of similar molecular weight (Fearon et al., 1974). Although both active and precursor factor D may be isolated by procedures which are designed to preserve the plasma proteins in their native state, e.g., gel filtration of plasma at neutral pH and physiological ionic strength in the presence of hexadimethrine and EDTA, the possibility that this low molecular weight factor may be a fragment of a larger serum protein precursor has not yet been excluded.

3.3. Control Proteins

The C1 inhibitor (C$\overline{1}$INH) has been highly purified and shown to be identical to the α2-neuraminoglycoprotein which had been isolated independently (Pensky and Schwick, 1969). As the latter name implies, this control protein contains a high percentage of carbohydrate, much of it neuraminic acid. The electrophoretic mobility of normal C$\overline{1}$INH is that of an α_2, but variations from this mobility have been observed in the sera of patients with the "genetic variant" form of C$\overline{1}$INH deficiency, in which an antigenically intact but non-functional C$\overline{1}$INH protein is inherited (Rosen et al., 1971). In two such kindreds, binding of the C$\overline{1}$INH to serum albumin has been found to account in part for the abnormal mobility. Whether the abnormal mobilities in others are attributable to differences in primary amino acid sequence or in carbohydrate composition is as yet unknown. In view of the dominant inheritance pattern which has been found, the latter seems a likely possibility.

The C3b inactivator (C3bINA) has been obtained in highly purified form (Ruddy et al., 1972b) but not in quantities sufficient for chemical studies. Inactivation of C3bINA by treatment with metaperiodate has been cited as evidence that carbohydrate residues are required for expression of the activity of this protein (Lachmann and Müller-Eberhard, 1968). Transferrin is usually the major contaminant in C3bINA preparations, and at one point it was incorrectly concluded that C3bINA and transferrin were the same protein (Torisu *et al.*, 1968). Antibody to C3bINA has been prepared, permitting its distinction from transferrin (Ruddy *et al.*, 1972*b*) and the identification of an inherited deficiency of C3bINA in a patient with hypercatabolism of C3, type-I (Alper *et al.*, 1972*c*).

4. REACTION MECHANISMS

4.1. General Principles

The phenomenon of *limited proteolysis* is central to the functioning of all of the plasma protein "effector systems"—including the coagulation, kinin-generating, fibrinolytic, complement, and properdin systems. The effects of complement activation are the consequence of a series of exquisitely specific and limited proteolytic reactions which catalyze the cleavage of certain of the complement proteins, the development of active enzymes from their precursors, and the formation of protein–protein complexes between two or more cleavage products. In the prototypal complement reaction (Fig. 1), the enzyme catalyzing the limited proteolysis has itself been activated either by a proteolytic reaction occurring earlier in the complement sequence or by a configurational change associated with its complexing to an appropriate activating agent. In general, cleavage of one or more specific peptide bonds in the substrate component liberates a minor fragment, which may have biologic activity; and a major fragment which is transiently capable of binding to a cell membrane or other appropriate surface. If binding occurs, it tends to stabilize the activity of the major fragment in forming a new enzyme or modifying the specificity of a preexisting enzyme, permitting the limited proteolysis of the next component in the sequence and continuing the series of complement reactions.

A second principle common to effector systems is that of *duplication*, i.e., the existence of two or more mechanisms which lead to similar effects. The

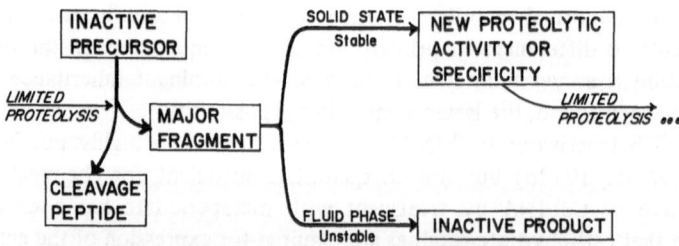

Fig. 1. The prototype of complement reactions.

several pathways leading to plasma enzymes which are capable of cleaving C3 are one example of such duplication; the formation during complement activation of factors chemotactic for leukocytes is a second; there are numerous others. Failure to appreciate the possibility of duplication was responsible for the eclipse of properdin research for a decade. Following the demonstration that some properdin preparations contained natural antibody to zymosan and that complexes of zymosan, antibody, and the first, fourth, and second components of complement could mimic the effects of zymosan and properdin in C3 destruction (Nelson, 1958), the existence of a separate, polysaccharide-activated pathway leading to the destruction of C3 was largely ignored. Research into the properdin system resumed only when sera congenitally deficient in C4 (May *et al.*, 1972) or C2 and antibody to the latter component (Marcus *et al.*, 1971) became available and provided conclusive evidence for the existence of a second pathway leading to C3 cleavage. It is now clear that, in normal serum under physiological conditions, both the classic and properdin systems contribute to the zymosan-induced inactivation of C3 (Gigli *et al.*, 1973) and that ablation of either system retards but does not completely block the inactivation reaction.

4.2. Classic Complement Activation

Human IgG of the IgG1, IgG2, and IgG3 subclasses and IgM appear to be capable of binding and activating the first component of complement. The complement-activating site, which is located on the Fc end of the H chain, not far from the hinge region, is apparent following aggregation of these immunoglobulins by heat or chemical crosslinking agents, or following union of immunoglobulin antibodies with their corresponding antigens. On the surface of sheep erythrocytes, a doublet of IgG molecules or a single IgM molecule is required for a C1-activating site (Borsos and Rapp, 1965). As a result of the binding of the C1 aggregate via its C1q subunit, the C1r portion becomes activated and acquires the capacity to activate C1s. Since trypsin and plasmin are also capable of activating C1s, and since $\overline{C1r}$ has demonstrable esteratic activity (Naff and Ratnoff, 1968), it seems likely that the activation of C1s involves its proteolytic cleavage by C1r. Activated $\overline{C1s}$, either as the free subunit or contained in the intact, activated $\overline{C1}$ molecule, cleaves its natural substrate, C4, into two fragments, the larger of which either becomes bound to the cell membrane to form the EAC14 complex (Borsos *et al.*, 1961) or remains free in the fluid phase as the inactive product C4i (Müller-Eberhard and Biro, 1963). The presence of C4b (or C4i) in a reaction mixture greatly enhances the activity of $\overline{C1}$ in cleaving its other natural substrate, C2 (Gigli and Austen, 1969). The major cleavage product of C2 joins with C4b in the formation of a magnesium-dependent protein–protein complex with new enzymatic activity, $\overline{C42}$, the classic C3 convertase (Müller-Eberhard *et al.*, 1967). This enzyme, whether present in the fluid phase or bound to the cellular intermediate EAC142, is unstable at 37°C; the addition of fresh C2 to EAC14 cells which have resulted from the decay of C2 from EAC142 regenerates $\overline{C42}$ and restores the C3-cleaving activity (Borsos *et al.*, 1961).

4.3. The Properdin System: Activation and Amplification

When zymosan is incubated with serum at 37°C, the C3 contained in the serum is inactivated to a much greater extent than are the C1, C4, and C2. This pattern of complement component utilization is distinctly different from that observed with classic complement fixation by immune complexes, in which the extent of utilization of C1, C4, and C2 greatly exceeds that of C3. The preferential utilization of C3 in the zymosan-induced reaction is attributable to activation of C3 via the properdin system, which includes both an activation pathway and an amplification or feedback loop (Fig. 2). Inulin, bacterial lipopolysaccharide, and certain other polysaccharides resemble zymosan in their ability to activate the properdin system, and at least some of these materials do so in the absence of detectable immunoglobulin (Gewurz *et al.*, 1970). Although aggregated human myeloma proteins of the IgG and IgM classes do not appear to activate this pathway, members of the IgA class are able to do so (Spiegelberg and Götze, 1972). The absence of a requirement for the classic activation system is readily demonstrable with serum from animals congenitally deficient in C2 or C4 or with serum rendered deficient by blocking the activity of C2 with antibody to this component. Kinetic differences between results obtained with

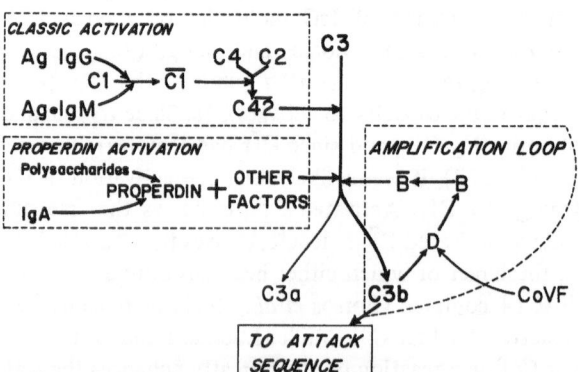

Fig. 2. Pathways leading to activation of C3 and the terminal complement sequence.

deficient and normal sera indicate an important contribution of the classic pathway in the normal serum reaction with zymosan, but C3 inactivation eventually proceeds to completion in the absence of C4 or C2.

As originally described, the properdin system (Pillemer et al., 1954), comprised of the serum factors required for the preferential inactivation of C3 by zymosan, included properdin, a protein which binds to zymosan at 17°C and can then be eluted by changes of pH and ionic strength; a heat-labile factor B (Blum et al., 1959); and a hydrazine-sensitive factor A (Pensky et al., 1959). Properdin itself, a 186,000 mol wt γ-globulin, appears to be involved in an activation sequence which parallels that of C1, C4, and C2. When purified from starting materials prepared by either elution from zymosan, euglobulin precipitation, or affinity chromatography with monospecific antiproperdin, properdin appears to be in an activated state; when the isolated properdin is reintroduced into fresh serum, cleavage of C3 ensues (Minta and Lepow, 1973). If purified C3 and properdin are incubated together, however, no C3 cleavage is observed, indicating a requirement for additional serum factors (Götze and Müller-Eberhard, 1973). The isolation of a serum protein of 70,000 mol wt which, in the presence of purified and activated properdin, leads to a direct attack on purified C3 has been reported (Spitzer and Stitzel, 1973). An alternative hypothesis, that activated properdin complexes with native C3 and thereby renders it capable of triggering the formation of a C3 convertase from factor B, has also been advanced (Götze and Müller-Eberhard, 1973).

The mechanism by which C3b, the major fragment of the initial step in C3 cleavage, is itself capable of inducing the formation of additional C3-cleaving activity has been delineated by studies of the properdin factors, of the sera of patients congenitally deficient in C3 or C3b inactivator, and of the mechanisms of action of the low molecular weight anticomplementary factor in cobra venom (CoVF). The presence of C3b together with factor D, a 25,000 mol wt euglobulin, triggers the activation of factor B, a 100,000 mol wt β-pseudoglobulin, and the cleavage of this protein into a 70,000 mol wt γ-fragment and a 30,000 mol wt α-fragment (Götze and Müller-Eberhard, 1971). C3b, produced by classic $C\overline{42}$, by the factor B dependent C3 convertase, or possibly by other mechanisms, appears to be required for initiation of the amplification loop. Factor B cleavage is not observed after the introduction of zymosan or similar agents into serum congenitally deficient in C3 (Alper et al., 1972b) or serum depleted of C3 by immunoabsorption. Cobra venom factor appears to mimic the effect of C3b in triggering the amplification except that the activated factor B formed during the CoVF-induced reaction appears to be more stable than that induced by C3b (Hunsicker et al., 1973; Fearon et al., 1973a). Like $C\overline{42}$, the classic C3 convertase, the C3b-induced factor B dependent C3 convertase, C3b·B(D), is capable of cleaving additional C3 and initiating the terminal attack sequence. The similarity between these two enzymes extends to their decay and regeneration.

Just as C3-cleaving activity may be restored by the addition of fresh C2 to EAC14 cells produced by decay of C2 from EAC142, so also the factor B dependent C3 convertase on EAC43B(D) may be regenerated following its decay by the addition of fresh factor B (Fearon *et al.*, 1973*b*).

4.4. The Terminal Sequence

Activation of the terminal attack sequence involves the proteolysis of two components, C3 and C5, and the subsequent assembly, through interactions which do not appear to be enzymatic, of a stable multimolecular complex comprised of C5, C6, C7, C8, and C9 (Kolb *et al.*, 1972) (Fig. 3). Although fluid-phase C3 convertase is capable of initiating these reactions and the formation of a fluid-phase hemolytically inactive C5–C9 complex is demonstrable, a cell-bound position for C3 convertase, as on EAC142, favors the deposition of the cleavage products C3b and C5b on the cell surface and the assembly of C5–C9 in the membrane in a cytolytically active form.

The cleavage of C3 by C3 convertase is a limited proteolytic reaction typical of the complement system (Fig. 1). A 7200 mol wt peptide, C3a, is released, and the major fragment, C3b, either binds to the cell surface or remains in the fluid phase as the inactive product, C3i. C3b modifies the substrate specificity of activated convertase, rendering it capable of cleaving C5. C5b, the larger of the two fragments produced by C5 cleavage, interacts with C6 to form C$\overline{56}$ (Thompson and Lachmann, 1970; Goldman *et al.*, 1972) and to begin the assembly of the multimolecular C5–C9 complex. Reaction of cell-bound C$\overline{56}$ with C7 leads to the formation of C$\overline{567}$, which is transiently capable of binding directly to the surface of cells which have not reacted with antibody or the earlier complement components. Cells bearing C$\overline{567}$ interact with C8, and then with C9, completing formation of the membrane-damaging complex, C5–C9. Although uptake of as

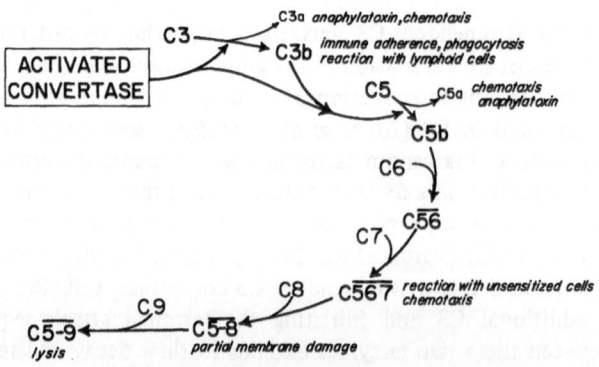

Fig. 3. The terminal complement sequence.

many as six molecules of C9 by a single C5–C8 complex is demonstrable, studies of the statistics and kinetics of the C9 step indicate that a single molecule of C9 suffices to prepare the cell for lysis (Ruddy et al., 1971).

4.5. Control Mechanisms

It is naive to view the complement and properdin systems as proteolytic cascades which, once activated, proceed inexorably to their final cytotoxic conclusion. Certain modulating influences are inherent in the reactions themselves: the rapid decay at 37°C of C̄42 and that of the factor B dependent C3 convertase are examples of inherent control mechanisms. Other retarding influences are the result of the natural inhibitors or inactivators, serum proteins which combine with or destroy enzymatically the activated forms of certain of the components.

4.5.1. C̄1 Inhibitor

C̄1 inhibitor blocks the activity of C̄1 or C̄1s, and has no effect on the precursor form of C1 which normally exists in serum. C̄1 bound to cellular intermediates, EAC1 and EAC14, is as susceptible to inhibition as is fluid-phase C̄1 (Lepow and Leon, 1962). The amount of C̄1 which is inhibited is independent of the initial concentration of C̄1, and during their interaction both C̄1 and C̄1INH are stoichiometrically depleted from the fluid phase (Gigli et al., 1968). Binding of labeled ^{125}I-C̄1s to C̄1INH in normal serum has been demonstrated (Rosen et al., 1971). The mechanism of action of C̄1INH therefore appears to involve its stoichiometric combination with C̄1, on or near its active site, so as to form an inactive complex.

4.5.2. C3b Inactivator

C3b inactivator, which appears to exist in serum or plasma in its active form, has no effect on native, fluid-phase C3. Its activity is readily demonstrable, however, when C3b has been bound to the cellular intermediate to form EAC1423 (Tamura and Nelson, 1967; Ruddy and Austen, 1969). The inactivation of the cell-bound C3b is time and temperature dependent, and C3bINA is not depleted from the fluid phase during the reaction, suggesting an enzymatic action of C3bINA. Studies with ^{125}I-C3 have demonstrated cleavage of C3b into two fragments, C3c (approximate mol wt 150,000) and C3d (approximate mol wt 30,000). In the case of cell-bound C3, C3c is released into the fluid phase and C3d remains bound to the cell surface. In the case of fluid-phase C3b, a similar cleavage reaction occurs. The mechanism of action of C3bINA is shown diagrammatically in Fig. 4 (Ruddy and Austen, 1971).

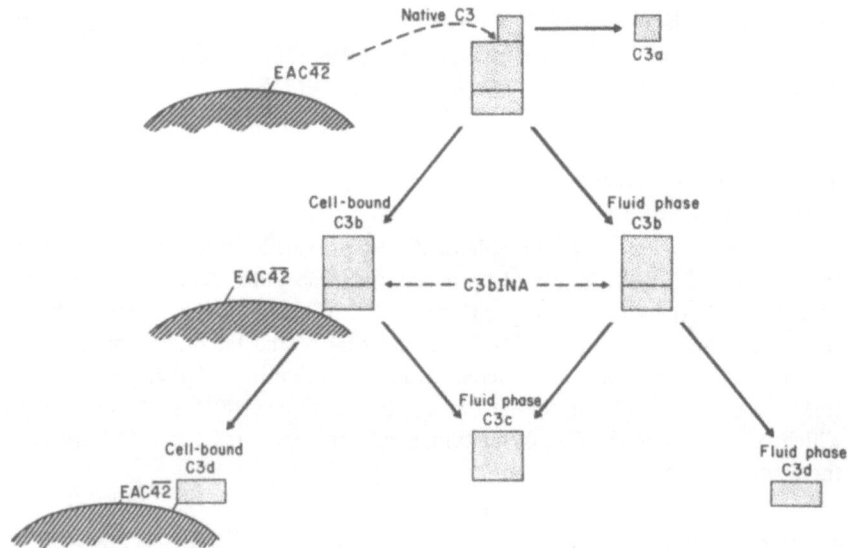

Fig. 4. Cleavage of C3 and its fragments.

C3bINA blocks all of the known biological effects of C3b, including the capacity to promote continuation of the hemolytic sequence, the enhancement of phagocytosis by leukocytes, and the immune adherence phenomenon. Most importantly, perhaps, C3bINA completely blocks the capacity of C3b to interact with factors D and B, in the formation of the factor B dependent properdin pathway C3 convertase (Ruddy *et al.*, 1973). C3bINA thus serves to oppose the positive feedback loop in which these factors participate. In a patient with C3 hypercatabolism, type I, unopposed cycling of this loop occurs, with circulating C3b (and no C3c), depressed levels of factor B, cleaving activity for factor B, and depressed levels of C3 present in the plasma (Alper *et al.*, 1972c). The C3bINA is therefore a control protein relating to both the classic complement and properdin pathways.

The anaphylatoxin inactivator is discussed in Section 5.1.2.

5. BIOLOGICAL ACTIVITIES

5.1. Permeability Factors

5.1.1. "C Kinin"

Evidence for the release, during activation of the classic pathway, of a peptide with permeability-enhancing properties is largely indirect, and comes from studies of the pathogenesis of the edema in patients with congenital C$\overline{1}$INH deficiency, or hereditary angioedema (Lepow, 1971). During attacks of edema, sera from patients contain activated $\overline{C1}$ (Donaldson and Rosen, 1964) and profoundly reduced serum levels of the natural substrates of this enzyme, C4 and C2 (Austen and Sheffer, 1965); C3 levels are usually within the normal range (Ruddy et al., 1968). Intradermal injection of $\overline{C1}$s into patients with $\overline{C1}$INH deficiency produces local attacks of edema resembling in appearance the edema which occurs spontaneously with attacks. Intradermal injection of $\overline{C1}$s into normal subjects produces a wheal, not blocked by antihistaminics, and requires the presence in vivo of C2 but not C3 (Klemperer et al., 1968). In vitro incubation of serum from patients with $\overline{C1}$INH deficiency generates a kinin-like peptide which contracts the isolated rat uterus but is clearly distinct from bradykinin. Generation of this peptide is inhibited by treatment of the serum with anti-C4 or anti-C2 but not anti-C3 (Donaldson et al., 1969). Evidence from both in vivo and in vitro experiments thus indicates that the interaction of $\overline{C1}$ with C4 and C2 is involved in the genesis of a material which locally increases vascular permeability.

Attempts to generate such a material by exposure of purified C4 and/or C2 to $\overline{C1}$ have met with limited success. The cleavage fragment, C4a, released during proteolysis of C4 by $\overline{C1}$ has some contractile activity on the rat uterus when used in high concentrations, but it is clearly not the peptide involved in the edema of $\overline{C1}$INH deficiency. A heat-stable peptide with physical and chemical properties similar to those of the peptide derived from incubation of $\overline{C1}$INH-deficient serum has been generated by the incubation of $\overline{C1}$ with C4 or with C2, or by trypsin treatment of C2, but the reliability with which the peptide is obtained is at present poor (Lepow, 1971). The hypothesis that "C-kinin," the pathogenetic peptide in hereditary angioedema, is a cleavage product of C2 currently awaits direct and definitive proof.

5.1.2. Anaphylatoxins

The cleavage peptides, C3a and C5a, are both anaphylatoxins; i.e., they cause release of histamine from mast cells, contract the guinea pig ileum with tachyphylaxis (the gut quickly becomes unresponsive to repeated stimulation with a given anaphylatoxin), and cause a local wheal when injected intracutaneously.

Any of a number of proteolytic enzymes, including $\overline{C42}$, the C3b-induced or CoVF-induced factor B dependent C3 convertase, trypsin, and plasmin, appear to be capable of cleaving C3a from the C3 parent molecule (Bokish et al., 1969); treatment of C3 with hydroxylamine also releases C3a. The especially labile peptide bond hydrolyzed in these reactions appears to contain an arginine and to occur approximately 60 amino acid residues from the N-terminal serine of one of the chains of C3. The anaphylatoxin C3a thus liberated has a molecular weight of 7800 with a C-terminal arginine and an N-terminal serine (Budzko et al., 1971). It is active in concentrations of 10^{-8} M on the guinea pig ileum and 2

$\times 10^{-12}$ M when injected into human skin, where it causes local edema and the degranulation of mast cells (Lepow *et al.*, 1970).

C5a may be cleaved from C5 by the classic enzyme $C\overline{423}$, by the factor B dependent convertase, or by trypsin (Cochrane and Müller-Eberhard, 1968). Its molecular weight appears to be approximately 15,000, and like C3a its activity depends on a C-terminal basic amino acid (see below). Although it has properties similar to those of C3a, C5a has different biological specificity. A guinea pig ileum made unresponsive to C3a by repeated stimulation with this peptide remains responsive to C5a; the converse is also true.

Although both C3a and C5a are readily produced by digestion of purified C3 and C5, the formation and the activity of both of these basic polypeptide cleavage products are difficult to demonstrate in whole human serum because of the presence of an anaphylatoxin inactivator. This enzyme, an α-globulin of approximately 310,000 mol wt, abolishes the biological activity of both C3a and C5a. In the case of C3a, release of the C-terminal arginine is associated with loss of activity. The serum anaphylatoxin inactivator resembles pancreatic carboxypeptidase B in its requirement for metal ions and its catalysis of the cleavage of C-terminal arginine or lysine residues, which appear to be essential for the biological activity of both C3a and C5a (Bokisch and Müller-Eberhard, 1970).

5.2. Chemotactic Factors

The first of the three complement-derived chemotactic factors to be described was C567 (Wards *et al.*, 1966), the multimolecular complex of C5, C6, and C7 which appears in the fluid phase during activation of the terminal sequence either by $C\overline{423}$ or by the C3b- or CoVF-induced factor B dependent enzymes. Although nascent $C\overline{567}$ has the capacity to attach to cell membranes, rendering these cells susceptible to lysis by C8 and C9 (Goldman *et al.*, 1972), this property of $C\overline{567}$ rapidly decays, leaving the chemotactic C567 complex (Lachmann *et al.*, 1970a).

Both of the cleavage peptides, C3a (Ward, 1967) and C5a (Ward and Newman, 1969), have been found to have chemotactic activity, the latter being considerably more active in most systems. In addition to the enzymes intrinsic to the complement and properdin systems which catalyze the formation of C3a and C5a, a variety of other proteases produce chemotactic factors from C3 and C5. In the case of C3, plasmin, trypsin, and a tissue protease present in most normal tissues produce a chemotactic fragment from C3. For C5, both trypsin and a neutral protease present in the lysosomal granules of polymorphonuclear leukocytes generate chemotactically active cleavage products. None of these fragments has been precisely characterized, relatively crude trypsin digests of purified C3 or C5 being used in most studies of complement-derived chemotactic factors. C5a is not only chemotactic but can also provoke the release of lysosomal enzymes into phagocytic vacuoles or the surrounding medium of polymorphonuclear leukocytes (Goldstein et al., 1973).

Although neutrophilic polymorphonuclear leukocytes were the first cell type shown to have a chemotactic response to complement-derived factors, eosinophils (Kay, 1970) and mononuclear leukocytes (Snyderman et al., 1971) have subsequently been shown to respond in a similar fashion. In the case of the polymorphonuclear cell, C567, C3a, and C5a appear to operate via a similar mechanism. Exposure of the cell to any one of these chemotactic factors renders it unresponsive or "deactivates" it for all of the others. Leukocytes which have been deactivated by exposure to C567, C5a, or C3a are also unresponsive to other chemotactic stimuli, such as bacterial filtrate. Activation of an identical intracellular serine esterase appears to be an initial step in the chemotactic response common to all three of the complement-derived chemotactic factors (Ward and Becker, 1968).

5.3. Adherence Phenomena

Immune complexes to which complement has become bound adhere to formed elements in the blood and in the reticuloendothelial system. In the phenomenon termed "immune adherence" (Nelson, 1953), such complexes were shown to adhere to primate erythrocytes and to nonprimate platelets. Binding of complement-coated complexes to polymorphonuclear leukocytes, to mononuclear cells, and to B-lymphocytes also occurs in most species which have been studied. These binding reactions may have important biological consequences, depending on the cell type involved (Henson, 1972).

5.3.1. Requirements for Adherence

Although immune adherence of sheep erythrocytes coated with C4 (EAC4) has been demonstrated for cells bearing high multiplicities of C4 (Cooper, 1969), in most cases the binding reactions appear to depend on the presence of a fragment of C3 on the surface of the immune complex. Thus EAC142 cells do not adhere, but EAC1423 cells, bearing the C3b fragment of C3, bind to human erythrocytes and certain other cells (Gigli and Nelson, 1968). Treatment with C3bINA, which cleaves C3c from the EAC1423 cell, leaving bound C3d, abolishes the immune adherence reaction, and this inhibition of immune adherence forms the basis for a useful functional assay for C3bINA (Ruddy and Austen, 1970). The immune adherence reaction appears to be uninfluenced by the presence or absence of components other than C3 on the immune complex, and, in fact, C3b which has been passively absorbed to tanned sheep erythrocytes serves to support the reaction (Okada et al., 1970).

Adherence of complement-coated complexes to human erythrocytes occurs over a wide range of pH. Most immune adherence reactions are temperature dependent and occur in the absence of divalent cations. In the case of adherence of immune complexes to rabbit neutrophils, however, the reaction is inhibited by EDTA, and agglomerates of neutrophils and adherent complexes are disrupted by treatment with this chelating agent (Henson, 1972).

The C3b receptor, present on the cells to which the immune complex adheres, has been shown to be trypsin sensitive and in this respect differs from the IgG receptor present on many of the same cells. Attempts to solubilize the immune adherence receptor site by treating human erythrocyte membranes with papain and pronase have met with limited success, and a material which, when present in the fluid phase, inhibits the adherence of EAC1423 to human E has been isolated (Nelson and Uhlenbruck, 1967).

Neutrophils and monocytes of all species studied have receptors for complement-coated complexes. Mouse and human B-lymphocytes also undergo adherence reactions with complement-coated complexes. Although platelets from nonprimate species (e.g., rabbit) appear to participate in immune adherence reactions, those from man and other primates do not. The reverse is true for erythrocytes: primate red cells have an immune adherence receptor, but those of nonprimate origin do not (Nelson, 1953; Henson, 1969).

5.3.2. Adherence to Phagocytic Cells

Binding of complement-coated immune complexes to monocytes or polymorphonuclear leukocytes promotes the phagocytosis of these complexes. The complement components required for enhancement of erythrocyte phagocytosis by polymorphonuclear leukocytes have been shown to be identical to those required for immune adherence to primate erythrocytes (Gigli and Nelson, 1968). Factors such as ionic strength of the medium, pH, and temperature have parallel effects on immune adherence and phagocytosis. By poisoning a serine esterase of the phagocyte, however, the binding of immune complexes can be dissociated from their subsequent engulfment (Pearlman *et al.*, 1969). Treatment of EAC43 cells with C3bINA abolishes their reactivity in phagocytosis, indicating that the presence of active C3b on the surface of the immune complex is required for the reaction.

In the case of certain polysaccharide antigens, C3b bound as a result of activation of the properdin system serves to enhance phagocytosis. Engulfment of pneumococci is promoted by both C4-deficient guinea pig serum and C2-deficient human serum, demonstrating the absence of a requirement for an intact classic activation pathway (Winkelstein *et al.*, 1973). Two additional factors, characterized as a heat-labile 5—6S β-pseudoglobulin and a dialyzable substance, were described as required for restoration of *in vitro* systems utilizing purified components to the full potency observed with unfractionated serum (Johnston *et al.*, 1969). These may have been properdin factor B and properdin factor D, respectively. The phagocytosis of endotoxin-containing oil droplets was also promoted by both C4- and C2-deficient serum, but neonatal cord serum, deficient in factor B, had diminished opsonic activity, which was restored by the addition of factor B; C3-deficient serum failed to opsonize the emulsion, and purified C3 restored this defect (Stossel *et al.*, 1973). The release of lysosomal enzymes consequent to the phagocytic process is discussed in detail in Chapter 1.

5.3.3. Platelet Adherence

Immune complexes or zymosan particles coated with C3b bind to platelets of certain species, including both rabbit and guinea pig but not human. As a consequence of this adherence, release of intracellular constituents such as nucleotides and vasoactive amines occurs, with acceleration of the coagulation process. The release reaction does not involve lysis of the platelet and requires calcium, energy metabolism, and the activity of a DFP-sensitive serine esterase contained in the platelet (Henson, 1972).

A second mechanism for the induction of platelet release, which occurs in the presence of high concentrations of immune complexes and complement and involves the cytolysis of the platelet, has also been described (Henson, 1970, 1972). In this system, intimate contact between the platelets and the immune complexes, induced by the C3b-dependent adherence, may result in the generation of active $\overline{C567}$ in the nearby fluid phase which, for a short time, is capable of binding to the platelet membrane, targeting it for destruction by C8 and C9. This "innocent bystander" cytolysis of platelets probably accounts for the acceleration of coagulation observed in whole rabbit blood following the introduction of immune complexes or properdin-activating polysaccharides (Zimmerman and Müller-Eberhard, 1971). This acceleration is not observed with blood from rabbits congenitally deficient in C6, and it is restored by the addition of purified C6. Presumably the C6-deficient blood is unable to generate $\overline{C567}$.

In contrast to the observations in rabbits, the addition of endotoxin or inulin to human blood from normal individuals or from a patient with homozygous C6 deficiency was found to have no consistent effect on the clotting time or prothrombin consumption (Leddy *et al.*, 1973). The difference in responses of human and rabbit blood may reflect the presence of the C3b-binding site on the platelets of only the latter species.

5.3.4. Adherence to Lymphocytes

Bone marrow—derived lymphocytes (B-cells) are distinguishable from thymus-derived lymphyocytes (T-cells) by their relatively large amounts of surface immunoglobulin, and membrane receptors for IgG or C3b contained in immune complexes (Dukor *et al.*, 1971). The capacity to form rosettes with sheep erythrocytes coated with antibody and complement has been used as a marker of B-cells or complement receptor lymphocytes. Studies with sheep cells coated with C3 by different methods have demonstrated that normal peripheral lymphocytes have two different kinds of receptors for C3. One appears to be specific for C3b, and in this sense identical to the receptors on phagocytic cells or primate erythrocytes; the second recognizes C3b which has been cleaved by C3b inactivator, and is presumably specific for the C3d fragment (Ross *et al.*, 1973; Eden *et al.*, 1973). The latter specificity, apparently unique to lymphocytes among cells, is also found on the bovine serum protein, conglutinin. In some studies, C3bINA has been termed "conglutinogen-activating factor," because of its capacity to render cells coated with C3b reactive with conglutinin (Lachmann and Müller-Eberhard, 1968). Although normal lymphocytes and cultured lymphoblastoid cells appear to have both kinds of receptors, lymphocytes from patients with chronic lymphatic leukemia, a neoplasm of B-cell origin, have receptors only for C3bINA-treated C3. A receptor for native C3 as well as for C3b has also been found on certain cultured lymphoma (RaJi) cells (Bokisch and Theofilopoulos, 1973). Binding of C3b to the RaJi cells and their subsequent exposure to fetal calf serum were associated with cytolytic destruction of the cells. This may be an instance in which C3b, bound to a membrane via an immune adherence receptor, triggered the formation of a factor B dependent convertase with consequent activation of C3 and the terminal ($C5$–$C9$) cytolytic sequence on the cell surface. The functions, if any, of the lymphocyte receptors for C3 and its fragments are as yet unknown, but evidence suggesting a role in B-cell activation has been reported.

5.4. Membrane Damage

5.4.1. Target Cells

The hallmark of complement action is the cytolytic destruction of cell membranes. Although most investigations of this phenomenon have been conducted with erythrocytes, studies with bacteria (Muschel and Treffers, 1956) and nucleated cells (Green *et al.*, 1959) have demonstrated that membranes of these cells are also susceptible to complement-induced damage. Even liposomes, artificial bilayer structures formed *in vitro* from known combinations of phospholipids and glycolipids, may be lysed by complement (Haxby *et al.*, 1969; Lachmann *et al.*, 1970*b*). Since these structures can be formed in the absence of protein, their susceptibility to lysis by complement excludes one of the theoretical mechanisms for this lysis, that the role of complement is to activate a membrane-bound enzyme which then catalyzes the cell to destroy itself.

5.4.2. Electron Microscopic Observations

The appearance of characteristic membrane discontinuities has been shown to accompany the action of complement on erythrocytes, bacteria, and lipsomes. The size of the discontinuity varies with the complement source: it is 100–110 Å for human and 85–98 Å for guinea pig complement. Provided that conditions are adjusted so as to exclude multiplier effects at the $\overline{C42}$ and C3 steps, the number of lesions corresponds quite closely to that predicted by the one-hit theory of immune hemolysis (Humphrey and Dourmashkin, 1965). Although initial studies indicated that the action of all nine components was required for the formation of these lesions, a recent study has reported their appearance following the C5 step (Polley *et al.*, 1971). Resistance of the lesions to treatment with proteolytic enzymes and their disappearance on extraction of the membrane with nonaqueous solvents suggest that they are located in the lipid bilayer of the membrane.

5.4.3. Mechanism

Studies of ion flux indicate that the initial step of complement-induced damage is a loss of the usual homeostatic controls of this flux (Green *et al.*, 1959). When the cell imbibes sufficient salts and water, it swells and the large membrane discontinuities which result permit the release of the internal macromolecular cell constituents. The latter step, osmotic lysis, can be prevented by suspending the cells in a medium of high ionic strength.

Since complement is capable of generating lesions on liposomes, and inducing their subsequent lysis, an effect on one or more of the lipid constituents of the membrane seems likely. Evidence for lipolytic activity accompanying the action of one or more of the terminal components has been reported (Smith and Becker, 1968; DeLage *et al.*, 1973), but independent experimental support for these reports has not thus far appeared. Studies with purified components have not demonstrated an enzymatic activity in the complement sequence beyond the cleavage of C5 by $\overline{C423}$. The existence of a decamolecular complex consisting of C5, C6, C7, C8, and C9 has been inferred from studies of the binding of purified and radiolabeled components to cellular intermediates formed during the terminal steps of hemolysis. The model involves a trimolecular arrangement of C5, C6, and C7 which forms a binding site for a single C8 molecule which in turn furnishes binding sites for as many as six C9 molecules (Kolb *et al.*, 1972). Direct demonstration of such a complex of C5–C9 in the fluid phase of reactions initiated by either the classic complement or the properdin pathway has been reported (Kolb and Müller-Eberhard, 1973). Although this fluid-phase complex is hemolytically inactive, it is postulated that a similar complex bound to cell membranes is the damaging agent. The most attractive working theory of cytolysis by complement involves the formation and insertion into the lipid bilayer of the membrane of a complex, formed from C5–C9, possessing a ringlike or doughnut structure and resembling very much the lesions observed on electron microscopic studies. The exterior of the ring is comprised of the nonpolar portions of the component complex, associated with lipids of the membrane, and the polar interior of the complex serves as a tunnel allowing the free flux of salt and water which eventuates in osmotic lysis (Mayer, 1972).

6. REFERENCES

Alper, C. A., and Propp, R. P., 1968, Genetic polymorphism of the third component of human complement (C'3), *J. Clin. Invest.* 47:2181.

Alper, C. A., Boenisch, T., and Watson, L., 1972a, Genetic polymorphism in human glycine-rich beta-glycoprotein, *J. Exp. Med.* 135:68.

Alper, C. A., Colten, H. R., Rosen, F. S., Rabson, A. R., Macnab, G. M., and Gear, J. S. S., 1972b, Homozygous deficiency of C3 in a patient with repeated infections, *Lancet* 2:1179.

Alper, C. A., Rosen, F. S., and Lachmann, P. J., 1972c, Inactivator of the third component of complement as an inhibitor in the properdin pathway, *Proc. Natl. Acad. Sci.* 69:2910.

Alper, C. A., Goodkofsky, I., and Lepow, I. H., 1973, The relationship of glycine-rich β-glycoprotein to factor B in the properdin system and to the cobra factor–binding protein of human serum, *J. Exp. Med.* 137:424.

Arroyave, C. M., and Müller-Eberhard, H. J., 1973, Isolation of the seventh component of the C system from human serum, *J. Immunol.* 111:302 (abst.).

Austen, K. F., and Sheffer, A. L., 1965, Detection of hereditary angioneurotic edema by demonstration of a reduction in the second component of human complement, *New Engl. J. Med.* 272:649.

Austen, K. F., Becker, E. L., Borsos, T., *et al.*, 1968, Nomenclature of complement, *Bull. WHO* 39:935.

Bing, D. H., 1971, Purification of the first component of human complement by affinity chromatography on human globulin linked to Sepharose, *J. Immunol.* 107:1243.

Blum, L., Pillemer, L., and Lepow, I. H., 1959, The properdin system and immunity. XIII. Assay and properties of a heat-labile serum factor (factor B) in the properdin system, *Z. Immunitaetsforsch.* 118:349.

Boenisch, T., and Alper, C. A., 1970, Isolation and properties of a glycine-rich γ-glycoprotein of human serum, *Biochim. Biophys. Acta* 214:135.

Bokisch, V. A., and Müller-Eberhard, H. J., 1970, Anaphylatoxin inactivator of human plasma: Its isolation and characterization as a carboxypeptidase, *J. Clin. Invest.* 49:2427.

Bokisch, V. A., and Theofilopoulos, A. N., 1973, Receptor for native C3 on human lymphoblastoid cell lines, *J. Immunol.* 111:300 (abst.).

Bokisch, V. A., Müller-Eberhard, H. J., and Cochrane, C. G., 1969, Isolation of a fragment (C3a) of the third component of human complement containing anaphylatoxin and chemotactic activity and description of an anaphylatoxin inactivator of human serum, *J. Exp. Med.* 129:1109.

Borsos, T., and Rapp, H. J., 1965, Hemolysin titration based on fixation of the activated first component of complement: Evidence that one molecule of hemolysin suffices to sensitize an erythrocyte, *J. Immunol.* 95:559.

Borsos, T., Rapp, H. J., and Mayer, M. M., 1961, Studies on the second component of complement. I. The reaction between EAC′1, 4 and C′2: Evidence on the single site mechanism of immune hemolysis and determination of C′2 on a molecular basis, *J. Immunol.* 87:310.

Brade, V., Cook, C., Shin, H., and Mayer, M. M., 1972, Studies on the properdin system: Isolation of a heat-labile factor from guinea pig serum related to a human glycine-rich beta-glycoprotein (GBG or factor B), *J. Immunol.* 109:1174.

Budzko, D. B., Bokisch, V. A., and Müller-Eberhard, H. J., 1971, A fragment of the third component of human complement with anaphylatoxin activity, *Biochemistry* 10:1166.

Cochrane, C. G., and Müller-Eberhard, H. J., 1968, The derivation of two distinct anaphylatoxin activities from the third and fifth components of human complement, *J. Exp. Med.* 127:371.

Cooper, N. R., 1969, Immune Adherence by the fourth component of complement, *Science* 165:396.

DeLage, J. M., Lehner-Netsch, G., and Simard, J., 1973, The tributyrinase activity of C7 *Immunology* 29:671.

Donaldson, V. H., and Rosen, F. S., 1964, Action of complement in hereditary angioneurotic edema: The role of C′1 esterase, *J. Clin. Invest.* 43:2204.

Donaldson, V. H., Ratnoff, O. D., Dias da Silva, W., and Rosen, F. S., 1969, Permeability-increasing activity in hereditary angioneurotic edema plasma. II. Mechanism of formation and partial characterization, *J. Clin. Invest.* 48:642.

Dukor, P., Bianco, C., and Nussenzweig, V., 1971, Bone marrow origin of complement-receptor lymphocytes, *Europ. J. Immunol.* 1:491.

Eden, A., Miller, G. W., and Nussenzweig, V., 1973, Human lymphocytes bear membrane receptors for C3b and C3d, *J. Clin. Invest.* 52:3239.

Fearon, D. T., Austen, K. F., and Ruddy, S., 1973a, Serum proteins involved in decay and regeneration of cobra venom factor–dependent complement activation, *J. Immunol.* 111:1730.

Fearon, D. T., Austen, K. F., and Ruddy, S., 1973b, Formation of a hemolytically active cellular intermediate by the interaction between properdin factors B and D and the activated third component of complement, *J. Exp. Med.* 138:1305.

Fearon, D. T., Austen, K. F., and Ruddy, S., 1974, Properdin factor D: Characterization of its active site and isolation of the precursor form, *J. Exp. Med.* 139:355.

Gewurz, H., Pickering, R. J., Snyderman, R., Lichtenstein, L. M., and Good, R. A., 1970, Interactions of the complement system with endotoxic lipopolysaccharides in immunoglobulin-deficient sera, *J. Exp. Med.* 131:817.

Gigli, I., and Austen, K. F., 1969, Fluid phase destruction of $C2^{hu}$ by $C1^{hu}$. I. Its enhancement and inhibition by homologous and heterologous C4, *J. Exp. Med.* 129:679.

Gigli, I., and Nelson, R. A., Jr., 1968, Complement dependent immune phagocytosis. I. Requirements for C′1, C′4, C′2, and C′3, *Exp. Cell. Res.* 51:45.

Gigli, I., Ruddy, S., and Austen, K. F., 1968, The stoichiometric measurement of the serum inhibitor of the first component of complement by the inhibition of immune hemolysis, *J. Immunol.* 100:1154.

Gigli, I., Koethe, S., and Austen, K. F., 1973, C3 destruction in serum by zymosan: Dependency on early components of complement and Hageman factor, *J. Immunol.* 111:288 (abst.).

Goldman, J. N., Ruddy, S., and Austen, K. F., 1972, Reaction mechanisms of nascent C$\overline{567}$ (reactive lysis). I. Reaction characteristics for production of EC567 and lysis by C8 and C9, *J. Immunol.* **109**:353.

Goldstein, I., Hoffstein, S., Gallin, J., and Weissmann, G., 1973, Mechanisms of lysosomal enzyme release from human leukocytes: Microtubule assembly and membrane fusion induced by a component of complement, *Proc. Natl. Acad. Sci.* **70**:2916.

Götze, O., and Müller-Eberhard, H. J., 1971, The C3 activator system: An alternate pathway of complement activation, *J. Exp. Med.* **134**:90s.

Götze, O., and Müller-Eberhard, H. J., 1973, The role of properdin in the alternate pathway of C activation, *J. Immunol.* **111**:288 (abst.).

Green, H., Barrow, P., and Goldberg, B., 1959, Effect of antibody and complement on permeability control in ascites tumor cells and erythrocytes, *J. Exp. Med.* **110**:699.

Haxby, J. A., Götze, O., Müller-Eberhard, H. J., and Kinsky, S. C., 1969, Release of trapped marker from liposomes by the action of purified complement components, *Proc. Natl. Acad. Sci.* **64**:290.

Henson, P. M., 1969, The adherence of leukocytes and platelets induced by fixed IgG antibody or complement, *Immunology (Lond.)* **16**:107.

Henson, P. M., 1970, Mechanisms of release of constituents from rabbit platelets by antigen antibody complexes and complement. I. Lytic and non-lytic reactions, *J. Immunol.* **105**:476.

Henson, P. M., 1972, Complement-dependent adherence of cells to antigen and antibody: Mechanisms and consequences, in: *Biological Activities of Complement* (5th International Symposium of the Canadian Society for Immunology, (D. G. Ingram, ed.), pp. 173–201, Karger, Basel.

Humphrey, J. H., and Dourmashkin, R. R., 1965, Electron microscope studies of immune cell lysis, in: *Ciba Foundation Symposium on Complement* (G. E. W. Wolstenholme and J. Knight, eds.), pp. 175–186, Churchill, London.

Hunsicker, L. G., Ruddy, S., and Austen, K. F., 1973, Alternate complement pathway: Factors involved in cobra venom factor (CoVF) activation of the third component of complement (C3), *J. Immunol.* **110**:128.

Inoue, K., and Nelson, R. A., Jr., 1965, The isolation and characterization of a new component of hemolytic complement C'3e, *J. Immunol.* **95**:355.

Inoue, K., and Nelson, R. A., Jr., 1966, The isolation and characterization of a ninth component of hemolytic complement, C'3f, *J. Immunol.* **96**:386.

Johnston, R. B., Klemperer, M. R., Alper, C. A., and Rosen, F. S., 1969, The enhancement of bacterial phagocytosis by serum, *J. Exp. Med.* **129**:1275.

Kay, A. B., 1970, Studies on eosinophil leukocyte migration. II. Factors specifically chemotactic for eosinophils and neutrophils generated from guinea pig serum by antigen–antibody complexes, *Clin. Exp. Immunol.* **7**:723.

Klemperer, M. R., Donaldson, V. H., and Rosen, F. S., 1968, Effect of C'1 on vascular permeability in man: Studies in normal and complement-deficient individuals and in patients with hereditary angioneurotic edema, *J. Clin. Invest.* **47**:604.

Kolb, W. P., and Müller-Eberhard, H. J., 1973, The membrane attack mechanism of complement: Veritifcation of a stable C5-9 complex in free solution, *J. Exp. Med.* **138**:438.

Kolb, W. P., Haxby, J. A., Arroyave, C. M., and Müller-Eberhard, H. J., 1972, Molecular analysis of the membrane attack mechanism of complement, *J. Exp. Med.* **135**:549.

Lachmann, P. J., and Müller-Eberhard, H. J., 1968, The demonstration in human serum of "conglutinogen-activating factor" and its effect on the third component of complement, *J. Immunol.* **100**:691.

Lachmann, P. J., Kay, A. B., and Thompson, R. A., 1970a, The chemotactic activity for neutrophil and eosinophil leukocytes of the trimolecular complex of the fifth, sixth, and seventh components of human complement (C567) prepared in free solution by the "reactive lysis" procedure, *Immunology* 19:895.

Lachmann, P. J., Munn, E. A., and Weissmann, G., 1970b, Complement-mediated lysis of liposomes produced by the reactive lysis procedure, *Immunology* 19:37.

Leddy, J. P., Frank, M. M., Gaither, T., Heusinkveld, R. S., Breckenridge, R. T., and Klemperer, M. R., 1973, Hereditary C6 deficiency in man, *J. Immunol.* 111:297 (abst.).

Lepow, I. H., 1971, Permeability-producing peptide byproduct of the interaction of the first, fourth and second components of complement, in: *Biochemistry of the Acute Allergic Reactions* (Second International Symposium, K. F. Austen and E. L. Becker, eds.), pp. 205–215, Blackwell Scientific Publications, London.

Lepow, I. H., and Leon, M. A., 1962, Interaction of a serum inhibitor of C'1-esterase with intermediate complexes of the immune haemolytic system. I. Specificity of inhibition of C'1 activity associated with intermediate complexes, *Immunology* 5:222.

Lepow, I. H., Naff, G. B., Todd, E. W., Pensky, J., and Hinz, C. F., 1963, Chromatographic resolution of the first component of human complement into three activities, *J. Exp. Med.* 117:983.

Lepow, I. H., Wilms-Kretschmer, K., Patrick, R. A., and Rosen, F. S., 1970, Gross and ultrastructural observations on lesions produced by intradermal injection of human C3a in man, *Am. J. Pathol.* 61:13.

Marcus, R. L., Shin, H. S., and Mayer, M. M., 1971, An alternate complement pathway: C3 cleaving activity, not due to C4, 2a, on endotoxic lipopolysaccharide after treatment with guinea pig serum; relation to properdin complement components, *Proc. Natl. Acad. Sci.* 68:1351.

May, J. E., Green, I., and Frank, M. M., 1972, The alternate complement pathway in cell damage: Antibody-mediated cytolysis or erythrocytes and nucleated cells, *J. Immunol.* 109:595.

Mayer, M. M., 1972, Mechanism of cytolysis by complement, *Proc. Natl. Acad. Sci.* 69:2954.

McLean, R. H., and Michael, A. F., 1973, Properdin and C3 proactivator: Alternate pathway components in human glomerulonephritis, *J. Clin. Invest.* 52:634.

Minta, J. O., and Lepow, I. H., 1973, Physical and chemical studies on human properdin purified by elution from zymosan and by affinity chromatography, *J. Immunol.* 111:286 (abst.).

Müller-Eberhard, H. J., 1961, Isolation and description of proteins related to the human complement system, *Acta Soc. Med. Upsal.* 66:152.

Müller-Eberhard, H. J., 1968, Chemistry and reaction mechanisms of complement, *Advan. Immunol.* 8:1.

Müller-Eberhard, H. J., and Biro, C. E., 1963, Isolation and description of the fourth component of human complement, *J. Exp. Med.* 118:447.

Müller-Eberhard, H. J., and Götze, O., 1972, C3 proactivator convertase and its mode of action, *J. Exp. Med.* 135:1003.

Müller-Eberhard, H. J., Polley, M. J., and Calcott, M. A., 1967, Formation and functional significance of a molecular complex derived from the second and the fourth component of human complement, *J. Exp. Med.* 125:359.

Müller-Eberhard, H. J., and Vallota, E. H., 1971, Formation and inactivation of anaphyla-toxins, in: *Biochemistry of the Acute Allergic Reactions* (2nd International Symposium, K. F. Austen and E. L. Becker, eds.), pp. 217, 242, Blackwell Scientific Publications, Oxford.

Muschel, L. H., and Treffers, H. P., 1956, Quantitative studies on the bactericidal actions of serum and complement. I. A rapid photometric growth assay for bactericidal activity, *J. Immunol.* **76**:1.

Naff, G. B., and Ratnoff, O. D., 1968, The enzymatic nature of C'1r: Conversion of C'1s to C'1 esterase and digestion of amino acid esters by C'1r, *J. Exp. Med.* **128**:571.

Nelson, D. S., and Uhlenbruck, G., 1967, Studies on the nature of the immune adherence receptor. I. The inhibition of immune adherence by soluble mucoids and mucopeptides and by human erythrocyte ghosts, *Vox Sang.* **12**:43.

Nelson, R. A., Jr., 1953, The immune adherence phenomenon: An immunologically specific reaction between microorganisms and erythrocytes leading to enhanced phagocytosis, *Science* **118**:733.

Nelson, R. A., Jr., 1958, An alternative mechanism for the properdin system, *J. Exp. Med.* **108**:515.

Nelson, R. A., Jr., 1966, A new concept of immunosuppression in hypersensitivity reactions and in transplantation immunity, *Surv. Ophthalmol.* **11**:498.

Nelson, R. A., Jr., Jensen, J., Gigli, I., and Tamara, R., 1966, Methods for the separation, purification, and measurement of the nine components of hemolytic complement in guinea pig serum, *Immunochemistry* **3**:111.

Nilsson, U., and Mapes, J., 1973, Polyacrylamide gel electrophoresis (PAGE) of reduced and dissociated C3 and C5: Studies of the polypeptide chain (PPC) subunits and their modifications by trypsin (TRY) and C42-C423, *J. Immunol.* **111**:293 (abst.).

Okada, H., Kawachi, S., and Nishioka, K., 1970, Immune adherence reactivity by C3 molecules without antibody and other factors of the complement system, *Biochim. Biophys. Acta* **208**:541.

Pearlman, D. W., Ward, P. A., and Becker, E. L., 1969, The requirement of serine esterase function in complement dependent erythrophagocytosis, *J. Exp. Med.* **130**:745.

Pensky, J., and Schwick, H. G., 1969, Human serum inhibitor of C'1 esterase: Identity with α2-neuraminoglycoprotein, *Science* **163**:698.

Pensky, J., Hinz, E. F., Jr., Todd, E. W., Wedgwood, R. J., Boyer, J. T., and Lepow, I. H., 1968, Properties of highly purified human properdin, *J. Immunol.* **100**:142.

Pensky, J., Wurz, L., Pillemer, L., and Lepow, I. H., 1959, The properdin system and immunity. XII. Assay properties, and partial purification of a hydrazine sensitive serum factor (factor A) in the properdin system, *Z. Immunitaetsforsch.* **118**:329.

Pillemer, L., Blum, L., Lepow, I. H., Ross, O. A., Todd, E. W., and Wardlaw, A. C., 1954, The properdin system and immunity. I. Demonstration and isolation of a new serum protein, properdin, and its role in immune phenomena, *Science* **120**:279.

Polley, M. J., and Müller-Eberhard, H. J., 1969, The second component of human complement: Its isolation, fragmentation by C'1 esterase, and incorporation into C'3 convertase, *J. Exp. Med.* **128**:533.

Polley, M. J., Müller-Eberhard, H. J., and Feldman, J. D., 1971, Production of ultrastructural membrane lesion by the fifth component of complement, *J. Exp. Med.* **133**:53.

Robbins, K. C., Summaria, L., Hsieh, B., and Shah, R. J., 1967, The peptide chains of human plasmin: Mechanism of activation of human plasminogen to plasmin, *J. Biol. Chem.* **242**:2333.

Rosen, F. S., and Alper, C. A., 1972, An enzyme in the alternate pathway to C3 activation and its inhibition by a protein in normal serum, *J. Clin. Invest.* **51**:80a (Abstract).

Rosen, F. S., Alper, C. A., Pensky, J., Klemperer, M. R., and Donaldson, V. H., 1971, Genetically determined heterogeneity of the C1 esterase inhibitor in patients with hereditary angioneurotic edema, *J. Clin. Invest.* **50**:2143.

Rosenfeld, S. I., Ruddy, S., and Austen, K. F., 1969, Structural polymorphism of the fourth component of human complement, *J. Clin. Invest.* **48**:2283.

Ross, G. D., Polley, K. J., Rabelline, E. M., and Grey, H. M., 1973, Two different complement receptors on human lymphocytes, *J. Exp. Med.* **138**:798.

Ruddy, S., and Austen, K. F., 1969, C3 inactivator of man. I. Hemolytic measurement by the inactivation of cell-bound C3, *J. Immunol.* **102**:533.

Ruddy, S., and Austen, K. F., 1970, Assay of C3 inactivator in biological fluids by inhibition of immune adherence of radioactive particles, *Fed. Proc.* **29**:433 (abst.).

Ruddy, S., and Austen, K. F., 1971, C3b inactivator of man. II. Fragments produced by C3b inactivator cleavage of cell-bound or fluid phase C3b, *J. Immunol.* **107**:742.

Ruddy, S., Carpenter, C. B., Müller-Eberhard, H. J., and Austen, K. F., 1968, Complement component levels in hereditary angioneurotic edema and isolated C'2 deficiency in man, in: *Mechanisms of Inflammation Induced by Immune Reactions* (Vth International Immunopathology Symposium, P. A. Miescher and P. Grabar, eds.), pp. 231–251, Schwabe, Basel.

Ruddy, S., Everson, L. K., Schur, P. H., and Austen, K. F., 1971, Hemolytic assay of the ninth complement component: Elevation and depletion in rheumatic diseases, *J. Exp. Med.* **134**:259s.

Ruddy, S., Gigli, I., and Austen, K. F., 1972a, The complement system of man, *New Engl. J. Med.* **287**:489, 545, 592, 642.

Ruddy, S., Hunsicker, L. G., and Austen, K. F., 1972b, C3b inactivator of man. III. Further purification and production of antibody to C3bINA, *J. Immunol.* **108**:657.

Ruddy, S., Fearon, D. T., and Austen, K. F., 1973, Participation of factors B, D, E, and C3b inactivator in cobra venom (CVF)-induced activation of the alternate C pathway, *J. Immunol.* **111**:289 (abst.).

Sakai, K., and Stroud, R. M., 1973, C1 proesterase (C1s): Purification, molecular properties and activation, *J. Immunol.* **111**:291 (abst.).

Smith, J. K., and Becker, E. L., 1968, Serum complement and the enzymatic degradation of erythrocyte phospholipid, *J. Immunol.* **100**:459.

Snyderman, R., Shin, H. S., and Hausman, M. H., 1971, A chemotactic factor for mononuclear leukocytes, *Proc. Soc. Exp. Biol. Med.* **138**:387.

Spiegelberg, H. L., and Götze, O., 1972, Conversion of C3 proactivator and activation of the alternate pathway of complement activation by different classes and subclasses of human immunoglobulin, *Fed. Proc.* **31**:2478.

Spitzer, R. E., and Stitzel, A. E., 1973, The properdin system: Identification of a factor activated by zymosan which interacts with properdin to convert C3, *J. Immunol.* **111**:212 (abst.).

Stossel, T. P., Alper, C. A., and Rosen, F. S., 1973, Serum-dependent phagocytosis of paraffin oil emulsified with bacterial lipopolysaccharide, *J. Exp. Med.* **137**:690.

Tamura, N., and Nelson, R. A., Jr., 1967, Three naturally occurring inhibitors of components of complement in guinea pig and rabbit serum, *J. Immunol.* **99**:582.

Thompson, R. A., and Lachmann, P. J., 1970, Reactive lysis: The complement-mediated lysis of unsensitized cells. I. The characterization of the indicator factor and its identification as C7, *J. Exp. Med.* **131**:629.

Torisu, M., Sonozaki, H., Shiraishi, S., and Nishioka, K., 1968, Purification of C'3 inactivator from human serum, *Nature (Lond.)* **218**:1163.

Valet, G., and Cooper, N. R., 1973, Isolation of the proenzyme forms of C1r and C1s from human serum, *J. Immunol.* **111**:292 (abst.).

Ward, P. A., 1967, Plasmin-split fragment of C'3 as a new chemotactic factor, *J. Exp. Med.* **126**:189.

Ward, P. A., and Becker, E. L., 1968, The deactivation of rabbit neutrophils by chemotactic factor and the nature of the activatable esterase, *J. Exp. Med.* **127**:693.

Ward, P. A., and Newman, L. J., 1969, A neutrophil chemotactic factor from human C'5, *J. Immunol.* **102**:93.

Ward, P. A., Cochrane, C. G., and Müller-Eberhard, H. J., 1966, Further studies on the chemotactic factor of complement and its formation *in vivo, Immunology* **11**:141.

Winklestein, J. A., Shin, H. S., and Wood, W. B., Jr., 1973, Heat labile opsonins to pneumococcus. III. The participation of immunoglobulin and the alternate pathway of C3 activation, *J. Immunol.* **108**:1681.

Yonemasu, K., and Stroud, R. M., 1971, C1q: Rapid purification method for preparation of monospecific antisera and for biochemical studies, *J. Immunol.* **106**:304.

Yonemasu, K., and Stroud, R. M., 1972, Structural studies on human C1q: Non-covalent and covalent subunits, *Immunochemistry* **9**:545.

Zimmerman, T. S., and Müller-Eberhard, H. J., 1971, Blood coagulation initiation by a complement mediated pathway, *J. Exp. Med.* **134**:1601.

HISTAMINE AND SEROTONIN

5

David A. Levy

1. HISTAMINE

1.1. Introduction

Histamine is an endogenous substance which is widely distributed in mammalian tissues. Although it has long been known to have potent biological actions, its role in various physiological and pathological phenomena has escaped precise definition. The strongest case can probably be made for its participation as a chemical mediator in inflammatory reactions. This chapter will review aspects of the structure and function of histamine which relate to its role as a mediator of inflammation. More extensive information is available in a number or books and monographs dealing with histamine and inflammation (Wolstenholme and O'Connor, 1955; Rocha e Silva, 1955, 1966; Spector and Willoughby, 1968; Kahlson and Rosengren, 1971; Zweifach *et al.*, 1973).

Histamine was first synthesized by Windaus and Vogt (1907) by the decarboxylation of histidine. Barger with Dale (1910) isolated from ergot (dried sclerotia of the fungus *Claviceps purpureo,* parasitic on rye plants) a base identified as histamine. Ackermann (1910) discovered that a similar base could

DAVID A. LEVY   Johns Hopkins Medical Institutions, Baltimore, Maryland

be isolated from putrefying mixtures containing histidine; histamine was produced in these mixtures by the decarboxylating action of bacteria. Barger and Dale also found histamine in intestinal mucosa, and Dale and Laidlaw (1910) noted its action on smooth muscle and blood pressure.

At the same time, there was much interest in acute anaphylactic reactions (Portier and Richet, 1902). Distinct differences were observed between anaphylaxis in dogs and that in guinea pigs. The actions of histamine in these two species resembled anaphylaxis sufficiently to suggest that the liberation of histamine might be responsible for at least some of the manifestations of that reaction. However, it was not until 1932 that the release of histamine in anaphylaxis was conclusively demonstrated (Bartosch *et al.*, 1932; Dragstedt and Gebauer-Fuelnegg, 1932).

In the intervening two decades, much attention was directed to the significance of histamine with regard to inflammation in general. For example, Eppinger (1913) observed that an injection of histamine into human skin produced a localized area of edema, a wheal. The extensive studies of Lewis and his colleagues indicated that a substance with the properties of histamine was released from cells in the skin by injurious stimuli, such as mild trauma and antigen–antibody interaction (Lewis, 1927). Interest in histamine was further stimulated by Dale in his Croonian lectures of 1929, and subsequently by Riley's discovery (1953) of the localization of histamine in mast cells. Recent advances in knowledge about histamine, mast cells, basophils, and immunological reactions make this an area of wide current interest.

1.2. Chemical Properties

Histamine, or 4-(2-aminoethyl)imidazole ($C_5H_9N_3$), has a molecular weight of 111, contains 37.8% nitrogen, and functions as a bivalent radical in salt formation. Its structure appears in Fig. 1. This basic substance is highly hygroscopic and very soluble in alcohol and hot chloroform; it is insoluble in ether and benzene. In aqueous solution, histamine base is rapidly destroyed by heating. In contrast, in acid solution it is stable even on prolonged boiling. The common salts of histamine are the dihydrochloride (184 mol wt) and the diphosphate (307 mol wt), which contain 64% and 36%, respectively, of the histamine base. It is necessary to consider these percentages when comparing effects of these salts with histamine base itself.

Histamine is produced commercially by bacterial decarboxylation of histidine and then is isolated either as the insoluble picrate or as the 3,4-dichlorobenzenesulfonate. The dihydrochloride salt is prepared from the latter with HCl in *n*-butanol; the diphosphate is prepared by treatment of the same salt with barium hydroxide followed by treatment with H_3PO_4.

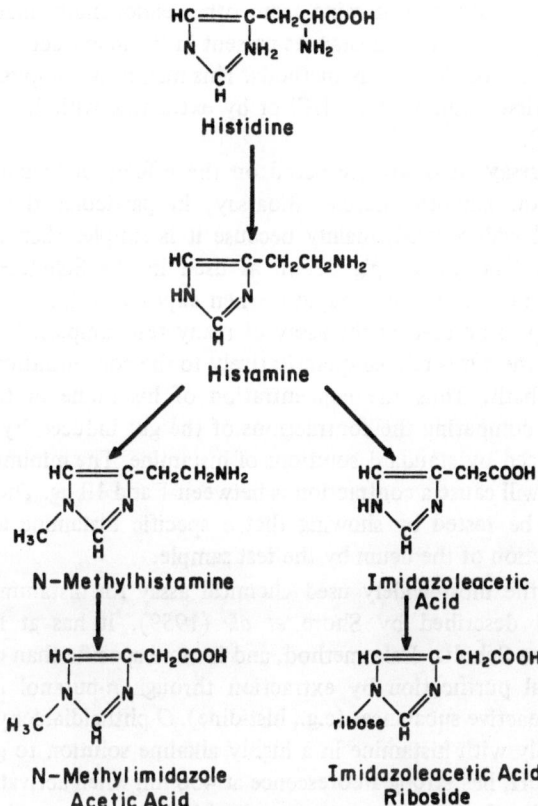

Fig. 1. Metabolism of histamine.

Free histamine crystallizes as colorless plates and melts at 83–84°C. It has no absorption maximum in the 210–700 nm region, nor does it exhibit fluorescence in the ultraviolet region. In aqueous solution, it has pK_a values of 5.94 and 9.80. It will form salts with several heavy metals, including silver, zinc, copper, and cobalt. It undergoes reactions characteristic of primary amines and of imidazole compounds, including acylation and diazotization. Precipitation as dipicrate and diflavinate salts, each of which has characteristic properties, has been used to identify histamine base in biological samples (Rocha e Silva, 1966).

1.3. Assay Methods

Histamine cannot be measured directly by photometric means. Therefore, it is determined either by bioassay or by chemical means (Rocha e Silva, 1966). In either case, separation of histamine from other endogenous pharmacologically active or chemically reactive substances present in tissue extracts and body fluids is required in some of these assay methods. This may be accomplished by boiling deproteinized tissue samples with HCl or by extracting with an organic solvent (e.g., n-butanol).

Biological assay methods are based on the effects of histamine on blood pressure and on smooth muscle. Bioassay, in particular the Schultz–Dale method, is still widely used, mainly because it is simpler than most chemical assay methods. The guinea pig ileum, as used in the Schultz–Dale method, contracts and then relaxes very rapidly when exposed to histamine, enabling a single ileal strip to be used in the assay of many test samples. The intensity of contraction of the gut is related quantitatively to the concentration of histamine in the tissue bath. Thus the concentration of histamine in test samples is determined by comparing the contractions of the gut induced by these samples and those induced by standard solutions of histamine. The minimum amount of histamine that will cause a contraction is between 1 and 10 ng. The specificity of the assay can be tested by showing that a specific histamine antagonist will prevent contraction of the ileum by the test sample.

Currently, the most widely used chemical assay for histamine is the fluorometric method described by Shore *et al.* (1959). It has at least as much sensitivity as the Schultz–Dale method, and is more specific than older chemical methods. Initial purification by extraction through n-butanol is required to remove other reactive substances (e.g., histidine). O-phthaldialdehyde (OPT) will condense rapidly with histamine in a highly alkaline solution to give a product which, at low pH, has strong fluorescence at 450 nm when activated at 350 nm. OPT reacts with other primary amines under highly alkaline conditions, but few of these compounds form an acid-stable fluorophore. Relative fluorescence of the OPT derivative of histamine is proportional to the initial histamine concentration over a wide range (5–500 ng/ml). The modification described by May *et al.* (1970) is recommended for use in studies with leukocytes and mast cells. OPT can also be used for the histochemical detection of cellular histamine in tissue sections and smears (Brody *et al.*, 1972).

Another method available for measurement of histamine is the enzymatic isotopic assay described by Snyder *et al.* (1966). This method depends on the enzymatic transfer of the methyl-^{14}C of S-adenosylmethionine-^{14}C to histamine to form methylhistamine-^{14}C. A tracer amount of histamine-^{3}H is added to the test sample. The final product formed is methylhistamine-^{14}C-^{3}H. The enzyme used for the reaction, histamine-N-methyltransferase, is highly specific for histamine; a crude salt extract of guinea pig brain serves as the enzyme in assay mixtures. No prior extraction of histamine from most tissue samples is necessary. Chloroform extraction separates methylhistamine from histamine. The radioactivity of the product is counted in a liquid scintillation counter; the ratio $^{14}C:^{3}H$ is linearly related to the content of histamine in the test sample. The percent of ^{3}H in this product indicates the extent of enzymatic methylation. A recent modification by Taylor and Snyder (1972) allows measurement of 0.1 ng or less histamine in 0.02 ml of tissue extract. This method has greater sensitivity and specificity than assays based on the preparation of other chemical derivatives, but it is somewhat more expensive to perform.

1.4. Distribution

Histamine is present in a wide variety of organisms, in which it appears to be a common constituent of secretions employed in attack and defense; for instance, it is a well-known component of bee venom. It is found in members of all vertebrate classes, from fish to mammals. Among vertebrates, mammalian tissues generally contain the greatest amounts of histamine. The histamine content of normal tissues varies with age, sex, species, and the season of the year; in inflammatory conditions, it may be increased or decreased. In mammals, histamine is distributed rather unevenly in various tissues, and its concentration in a tissue is related mainly to the number of mast cells in that tissue. In the blood of most mammals, histamine is present mainly in basophilic leukocytes; in rabbit blood, it is present largely in platelets. Large amounts of histamine are present in a non-mast-cell localization in the oxyntic gland area of the stomach. Significant amounts are present in both central and peripheral nervous tissues. Schayer (1965) and Kahlson and Rosengren (1971) have suggested that histamine is also present in cells other than mast cells, e.g., smooth muscle cells or vascular endothelial cells, in a form which they refer to as "induced" or "nascent" histamine. The existence of histamine in these forms is based only on indirect evidence.

In man, lungs, intestinal mucosa, and skin have a relatively high histamine content: lung about 20–30 μg histamine base/g wet tissue, duodenum about 15 μg histamine base/g wet tissue, and skin about 8 μg histamine base/g wet tissue. Since the skin comprises about 6% of the total body weight, there is about 30 mg histamine in the skin of an average-sized adult. Within an organ, the distribution of histamine may be uneven. For example, in guinea pig skin, histamine is most abundant around the ears, snout, eyelids, nipples, and perineum. Most of this is present in the dermis; the epidermis contains very little histamine. As expected, mast cells are most abundant in those areas of the skin which have the highest histamine content (Rocha e Silva, 1966).

Nearly all the histamine in human blood is limited to basophilic leukocytes, which normally comprise less than 0.5% of all the leukocytes. The histamine content of whole blood, or the leukocyte fraction thereof, normally ranges from

0.02 to 0.08 μg histamine base/ml, depending of course on the absolute basophil count. No significant difference has been noted in the histamine content of blood between allergic and nonallergic groups of individuals. Normally the basophil count, and therefore the histamine content of an individual's blood, varies little over time, but both may be significantly reduced shortly after an anaphylactic reaction and in persons receiving corticosteroids. The histamine content of plasma is normally below the limits of detection. Since large amounts of histamine are present in rabbit platelets, the serum may contain appreciable amounts of histamine.

Free mast cells can be isolated from the peritoneal cavity of a normal rat by washing this cavity with saline solution. Mast cells comprise about 5–10% of the total cells in the suspension, depending on the strain of the rat; about 10^6 mast cells can be obtained from a single rat's peritoneal cavity. There is about 10–15 μg histamine/10^6 rat mast cells. Mast cells can easily be identified in these suspensions after staining with 0.05–0.5% toluidine blue; they are cells with abundant purple-stained cytoplasmic granules. Other methods for staining mast cells are mentioned in Selye (1965). The metachromasia of mast cells and of basophils is due to the presence of heparin, a strongly anionic mucopolysaccharide, in the cytoplasmic granules. Heparin and protein (mainly proteases) account for over 95% of the dry weight of the granules. These granules are surrounded by a distinct perigranular membrane which is seen best by electron microscopy and which is regarded as an insulator against cytoplasmic ions. The granules themselves are electron dense and show varying degrees of amorphous, crystalline, and lamellar structures. Their main function appears to be to serve as intracellular storage sites for histamine and other biologically active components; under the influence of appropriate stimuli, mast cells and basophils are able to secrete these substances by an extrusive process involving fusion of perigranular membranes with plasma membrane.

1.5. *Metabolism*

Histamine is synthesized in mast cells and basophils from L-histidine by a specific cytoplasmic histidine decarboxylase, which requires pyridoxal-5-phosphate as a coenzyme. The enzyme can be inhibited by α-methylhistidine and 4-bromo-3-hydroxybenzyloxyamine (NSD-1055). DOPA decarboxylase can also decarboxylate histidine, but it may have little to do with histamine formation *in vivo*. It is also unlikely that exogenous histamine contributes to the pool of histamine in mast cells and basophils. The pathway of histamine from its presumed site of synthesis in the cytoplasm to its storage site in the granules is unknown. Once inside the granule, it appears to be retained there, possibly for many weeks, through firm ionic linkage to carboxyl groups on granule proteins.

Granules have been isolated intact without their perigranular membrane by lysis of rat mast cells in distilled water. Such free granules retain their histamine until they are exposed to a salt-containing solution, suggesting that the release of histamine from the granule matrix is probably a physicochemical event (i.e., an ion exchange process) which occurs immediately on exposure of the granule to cations in the extracellular medium (Uvnäs, 1967). The biological effects of histamine occur only after it has been released from its storage sites in mast cells and basophils. Release of histamine can be induced by a variety of stimuli, but there is no evidence that it is delivered into tissues or blood under normal circumstances, although this possibility has not been ruled out.

Once histamine has been released from the cell, its effects are fairly transient because it is rapidly converted to inactive derivatives (Fig. 1). Inactivation occurs by methylation of the ring imino-nitrogen to form N-methylhistamine followed by oxidation of the side-chain to form methylimidazoleacetic acid. The histamine-N-methyltransferase which catalyzes this reaction is present in many tissues. A second pathway proceeds by oxidation through imidazole-4(5)-acetaldehyde to imidazole-4(5)-acetic acid. This reaction is catalyzed by a diamino oxidase (histaminase) which is probably not specific for histamine; it is particularly abundant in kidney. Much of the imidazole acetic acid is conjugated with ribose and excreted in the urine as such. Study of the catabolism of histamine-^{14}C in man showed imidazoleacetic acid to be the principal metabolic product recovered in the urine (Beall and VanArsdel, 1960). Labeled imidazole-acetic acid riboside and methylimidazoleacetic acid were also recovered, but histamine-^{14}C itself was not detected. In other species, methylation appears to be the major catabolic pathway.

1.6. Pharmacological and Physiological Effects

The major pharmacological properties of histamine are regarded as (a) contraction of smooth muscle, (b) dilation of small blood vessels, and (c) stimulation of secretion from exocrine glands. The *in vivo* response to an injection of histamine varies in animals of different species for reasons which are not yet known. In gross terms, the response depends on which tissues in the animal are particularly sensitive to histamine and on the occurrence of secondary effects such as stimulation of the sympathetic nervous system. In cats and dogs, for example, 0.3 mg histamine/kg body weight given intravenously produces intense salivation, vomiting, diarrhea, dyspnea, and hypotension, followed by recovery within an hour. The same dose given to a guinea pig may be rapidly fatal due to sudden, marked airway obstruction leading to asphyxia and death. An i.v. dose of the same size in man produces a violent, pulsating headache with a sense of cranial compression, flushing of the face, and a slight tachycardia. Little change in blood pressure may be noted with this dose. Some subjects may experience nausea, vomiting, and diarrhea. Most of these symptoms last for only a few minutes. Larger doses may produce intense pruritus, especially on the face and hands, and flushing which is sometimes followed by urticaria on the upper body (Rocha e Silva, 1966).

The effect of histamine on smooth muscle can be demonstrated *in vitro*. Intestinal, bronchial, and uterine smooth muscle are particularly sensitive to it. However, the degree and type of response will vary depending on the source of the organ. For example, whereas guinea pig uterus contracts sharply when exposed to 10 ng histamine, rat uterus relaxes when exposed to a similar dose.

The most striking effects of an i.v. injection of histamine on the circulation (*viz.*, hypotension and edema) are a consequence of generalized vasodilatation which is secondary to contraction of endothelial lining cells in postcapillary venules, vessels whose diameters range from 20 to 30 μm. These cells normally form a closed cylinder within which blood flows. When the endothelial cells are caused to contract by histamine, they pull away from each other, producing gaps between adjacent cells. These discontinuities allow egress of plasma, fine particles, and platelets from the vascular lumen. Plasma then filters through the semipermeable periendothelial basement membrane and into surrounding tissue spaces, increasing extravascular fluid volume and simultaneously reducing intravascular volume; small particles and cells are retained by the basement membrane (Majno, 1965).

The flow of plasma into the perivascular space can be observed by initially labeling plasma proteins with a colored dye or with radioactive iodine. Evans blue dye, for example, forms a stable complex with albumin. If, after an i.v. injection of 0.5 ml of 0.5% Evans blue dye into a guinea pig, histamine is injected in a small volume into the animal's shaved skin, a small area of bluing will develop around the injection site as a result of the local increase in vascular permeability. The local reaction begins within 3–5 min after the injection of histamine, and it ceases to enlarge within 10–15 min. It can be shown that the area of leakage of plasma (i.e., the size of the colored spot in the skin) is directly proportional to the log dose of histamine. A more accurate measure of the response can be obtained by extracting the protein-bound dye that accumulates in the local site.

Effects on the circulation may also result from actions of histamine on the heart. Histamine increases the rate, the force of contraction, and the time of atrioventricular conduction of the heart by a direct stimulatory action on cardiac smooth muscle (Levi, 1972).

Histamine is regarded as having a physiological role in the stomach (Levine, 1968; Håkanson and Liedberg, 1971). Feeding and vagal stimulation cause the secretion of gastrin, which then induces the release of histamine from its specific non-mast-cell storage sites in the gastric mucosa. Histamine reaches parietal cells by diffusion and stimulates them to secrete HCl. Additionally, the release of histamine from its storage sites causes increased local activity of histidine decarboxylase, presumably to replenish the mucosal supply of histamine. The pharmacological action of histamine on the human stomach can be demonstrated by an i.v. infusion of 0.004 μg histamine/kg/min. This infusion produces a copious flow of gastric juice with high acidity and large amounts of pepsin (Rocha e Silva, 1966).

Histamine has less powerful stimulatory effects on other exocrine glands, such as salivary, lacrimal, bronchial, pancreatic, and intestinal mucous glands. It is probably not a major regulator of the physiology of these glands, but effects can readily be demonstrated with pharmacological doses of histamine.

As a result of recent research on cyclic adenosine 3',5'-monophosphate (cAMP) as an intracellular "second messenger" and on the control of cAMP by histamine and hormones, Bourne et al. (1974) have proposed that histamine, in concert with these other substances, acts in vivo to regulate the character and intensity of inflammatory and immune responses. They suggest that this regulation is mediated by the inhibitory action of cAMP on various types of leukocytes. Thus histamine released from mast cells by an antigen–antibody reaction or by trauma might act not only to produce immediate local inflammatory changes but also to limit the extent of inflammation by preventing release of mediators from cells at the edge of the initial reaction. This hypothesis, if confirmed, will extend present understanding of the role of histamine in the inflammatory process (infra vide).

1.7. Effect at a Cellular and a Molecular Level

The various biological effects of histamine are visualized as being mediated through its interaction with specific receptors located on the plasma membrane of cells in target tissues. Receptors for other pharmacologically active substances (e.g., epinephrine) are on the same cells. The histamine receptor on smooth muscle is said to contain a histidyl radical as part of its active center (Rocha e Silva, 1966). A large number of analogues of histamine have been synthesized for use in studies of its mechanism of action. Most compounds having histamine-like biological activities contain small nitrogen-heterocyclic aromatic rings to which are attached 2-aminoethyl side-chains. Certain of these analogues mimic histamine in only one of its pharmacological effects; for instance, they may stimulate gastric secretion but have little effect on smooth muscle. For example, 4-methylhistamine is more active as an agonist on rat gastric acid secretion, rat uterus, and guinea pig atrium than it is on guinea pig ileum or rat gastric smooth muscle. Such observations suggest that receptors for histamine in various tissues may differ in subtle ways. Support for the existence of more than one type of histamine receptor also comes from experiments showing that its effect on certain tissues (e.g., guinea pig ileum) can be antagonized by typical antihistamine compounds (e.g., mepyramine maleate), whereas the effect of histamine on other tissues (e.g., rat uterus) is not blocked by the same antihistamines. This led Ash and Schild (1966) to hypothesize two different types of histamine receptors: H_1-receptors, which are sensitive to the usual antihistamines (e.g., mepyramine), and H_2-receptors, which cannot be blocked by the same antihistamines. Proof for the existence of H_2-type receptors was recently provided by Black *et al.* (1972), who discovered two new compounds, burimamide or N-methyl-N'-[4-(4(5-imidazolyl)butyl] thiourea, and metiamide or N-methyl-N'-[(2(5)-methylimidazol-4-yl)methylthio)ethyl] thiourea, which act as specific histamine antagonists on rat gastric acid secretion, rat uterus, and guinea pig atrium, but do not inhibit the action of histamine on guinea pig ileum. Recent studies suggest that the heart and the peripheral vascular system may have both H_1- and H_2-type histamine receptors (Levi and Lee, 1974; Powell and Brody, 1974). Human leukocytes also have receptors for histamine (Melmon *et al.*, 1972), and these receptors have recently been identified as H_2-type receptors (Lichtenstein and Gillespie, 1973).

The intracellular events which follow the interaction of histamine and H_2-receptors are beginning to be documented. The addition of histamine to heart muscle and leukocytes is followed by an increase in the intracellular concentration of cAMP. The level of this compound in cells is controlled mainly by two enzymes, adenylate cyclase, which is associated with the plasma membrane and which catabolizes the formation of cAMP from ATP, and cAMP phosphodiesterase, a cytoplasmic enzyme, which hydrolyzes the phosphodiester bond of cAMP, converting it to $5'$-AMP. The interaction of histamine and H_2 membrane receptor leads to activation of adenylate cyclase. The mechanism by which changes in cAMP concentration are related to the observed effects of histamine (i.e., enhancement or inhibition of cell function) is unknown. Ultimately, these events may involve contractile elements within a variety of cells. At the present time, virtually nothing is known about the biochemical events which follow interaction of histamine with H_1-type receptors.

1.8. Role in Inflammation

1.8.1. Histamine Release

Histamine is the one chemical mediator for which a role in the mechanism of inflammation has clearly been established (Spector and Willoughby, 1968). Since the earliest response to various types of local injury is vasodilatation with an increase in vascular permeability, the known effects of histamine on the microvasculature qualify it for such a role in the early stages of inflammation. The concentration of histamine in tissue fluid at a site of local injury rises transiently within minutes following an insult, and the amount of histamine in the injured tissue is reduced thereafter. This reduction in histamine content is associated with an altered appearance (*viz.*, degranulation) of the mast cells in the injured tissues. In this regard, it is of interest that mast cells are most abundant around small blood vessels in connective tissues where inflammation is apt to occur. If tissue histamine stores are depleted by one means or another prior to the local injury, then the vascular response which usually occurs in the initial stages of an inflammatory response is significantly reduced. Furthermore, pre-medication with an antihistamine will also reduce the early vascular response to injury. In any case, the role of histamine in the inflammatory response is probably transient; other mediators and mechanisms are required to explain the continued vascular and cellular changes which develop as the response progresses and then regresses. Bourne's recent hypothesis (1974) may provide some of the answers.

Histamine can be released from its intracellular storage sites either through a secretory mechanism or by cytotoxic injury to cells containing it. In either case, once it is released into the extracellular milieu, effects noted above will follow. The specific type of tissue reaction which is then observed depends on a large number of factors, including the site of the release and the circumstances that induce it. Among the wide variety of agents which can induce histamine release are the following: antigens and antibodies; chemical, thermal, or mechanical injury; X-irradiation; peptides and proteins derived from plasma proteins, e.g., complement, and from blood cells; drugs such as codeine, morphine, and atropine; certain organic bases such as compound 48/80 and polymyxin B; venoms and toxins; surface-active agents such as tweens; and certain large molecules such as dextran. The remainder of this section will be concerned with certain inflammatory conditions for which there is evidence that histamine release is induced by immunological mechanisms, or in which mast cells and basophils appear to have a significant role.

1.8.2. The Allergic Reaction

The first of these conditions to be considered is the allergic, or immediate hypersensitivity, reaction. The term "allergy" was originally defined as a state of altered immunological reactivity to foreign substances. Now it is used to indicate certain pathophysiological changes caused by immunologically induced release of chemical mediators, among which are histamine, from tissue mast cells and circulating basophils. The clinical states which result, called "allergies" when they occur in humans and dogs, depend in part on the nature of the antigen, its site of entry, and the tissue in which it reacts with antibody as well as the quantities of antigen and antibody participating in the reaction. The commonly recognized allergies of man include allergic rhinitis, asthma (certain cases), urticaria (certain cases), and systemic anaphylaxis. In each of these conditions, at least part of the pathophysiological alteration can be explained by the pharmacological actions of histamine. The finding of a close correlation between antigen-induced histamine release from leukocytes *in vitro* and the magnitude of patients' symptoms in the hay fever season provides further evidence for the participation of histamine as a mediator of human allergic disease (Lichtenstein, 1972).

While most antigens that cause allergic reactions, sometimes referred to as "allergens," are proteins, allergic sensitivity may also exist to a variety of other substances including polysaccharides (e.g., dextrans) and haptens (e.g., penicillin). Clinically the most important are those causing pollinosis. These are protein components of the pollens of grasses, trees, and weeds. Their molecular weights are in the range of 30,000–40,000, and they can induce an immediate local reaction in a sensitized patient when as little as 10^{-14} to 10^{-15} g is injected intradermally. Other clinically important protein allergens are present in mold spores, animal danders, organic dusts, insect venoms, and foods.

When certain individuals encounter these allergens in nature, they respond by producing antibodies of several immunoglobulin classes, particularly IgE antibodies, which are also called "reaginic," "skin-sensitizing," or "anaphylactic" antibodies. Reaginic antibodies differ from antibodies of the other Ig classes primarily by their ability to bind firmly and for prolonged periods to the surface of mast cells and basophils. Cells to which specific reaginic antibody is bound are said to be "sensitized," and the individual having such cells is allergic to the allergen for which the antibody is specific. IgE antibodies are present in very low concentration (usually less than 1 µg/ml) in the serum of allergic individuals, which explains why they are not detectable by precipitation and agglutination tests. Their ability to passively sensitize the mast cells and basophils of a nonallergic individual is destroyed by mild heating (56°C for 1–4 h). The ability of IgE to sensitize these target cells is a property of the Fc portion of these molecules; it permits them to interact with specific receptors on these target cells. Immunoglobulin E, which has a molecular weight of about 200,000, is present in the serum of all normal individuals in very low concentration (0.1–0.7 µg/ml). In allergic individuals, specific IgE antibodies are synthesized in response to contact with very small quantities of antigen (e.g., less than 1 µg/yr in the case of pollen allergens). It is possible for almost everyone to produce detectable levels of IgE antibody, if given the appropriate antigen (e.g., an extract of the nematode *Ascaris*). However, only a limited proportion of the population, probably about 20%, develop allergies spontaneously. Why this should be the case is not known, but there is reason to believe that it is related not only to environmental factors (e.g., exposure to very low doses of allergen) but also to genetic factors (e.g., specific immune response genes).

Reaginic (IgE) antibodies have also been identified in the monkey, cow, sheep, pig, dog, rat, mouse, and guinea pig. Anaphylactic antibodies of the IgG type have been identified in the guinea pig (IgG1a), in the mouse (IgG1), and in the rat (IgGa), and there may be a similar antibody in man. These IgG antibodies have been induced by immunization with protein antigens and hapten—carrier complexes, and they tend to be present in serum in relatively high concentration, and resist inactivation by heating at 56°C. They react with mast cells of the same species and sensitize them for antigen-induced histamine release, which homologous antibodies of other Ig types (except IgE) do not do. However, the nature of their binding to mast cells is different from the binding of IgE to mast cells. In particular, the binding is much less firm, and, as a consequence, passive sensitization by IgG antibody persists for less than 4 days, whereas passive sensitization by IgE antibody may be detected for 4 wk or longer. Both antibodies require a latent period for maximum sensitization to occur; with IgG anaphylactic antibodies, the optimum latent period is 2—6 h, whereas with IgE antibodies, the optimum latent period is 24—72 h or longer (Bloch, 1973).

IgE molecules on the surface of mast cells and human basophils have been detected both microscopically and functionally with specific anti-IgE antiserum, prepared (in the case of human and rat IgE) with IgE purified from the serum of individuals with plasmacytosis, or multiple myeloma. There appear to be about 10,000—250,000 IgE molecules/cell. In allergic individuals, an unknown proportion of these molecules represents antibody specific for common allergens. In highly sensitive individuals, it appears that only a small number of allergen molecules, possibly about 100/cell, are required to cause histamine release. It has been suggested that for release to be triggered by allergen or by anti-IgE antibody the triggering molecule must bridge two cell-bound IgE molecules. As discussed previously, details concerning the subsequent intracellular processes which result in mediator release are not known, although it is clear that this is a secretory process that is modulated by intracellular cAMP and by extracellular hormones (e.g., epinephrine) which affect cAMP levels in the cell. The initial steps after antigen—antibody union on the cell surface may result in a transient decrease in cAMP concentration. Once these steps have occurred, release probably requires several additional steps which involve cytoplasmic microtubules, metabolic energy, and calcium ions.

Modulation of the release reaction can be demonstrated with hormones and drugs which are capable of changing intracellular cyclic nucleotide levels. Of particular interest is the observation that exogenous histamine at concentrations which are present in leukocytes can increase the cAMP level of these cells and inhibit the antigen-induced release of endogenous histamine (Lichtenstein, 1972). The rise in cAMP and inhibition of histamine release from basophils by histamine are not blocked by standard H_1-type antihistamines but are blocked by burimamide, an H_2-receptor antagonist (Lichtenstein and Gillespie, 1973).

These findings indicate that basophils (and probably mast cells, also) have H_2-type receptors. More recently, the H_2-receptor antagonist, metiamide, was shown to enhance IgE-mediated histamine release from lung fragments (Chakrin *et al.*, 1974), thus providing further evidence for a feedback mechanism modulating the function of cells in this acute inflammatory reaction.

Much of the pathophysiology of hypersensitivity reactions mediated by IgE antibodies can be explained on the basis of the pharmacological effects of histamine: acute vasodilatation and edema formation, increased mucus secretion, and smooth muscle contractions. In clinical situations, these ractions may persist for more than a matter of minutes, and this persistence may be explained in part by the simultaneous release of other mediators as well as by continued contact with the inciting allergen. Slow reacting substance of anaphylaxis (SRS-A) and eosinophil chemotactic factor of anaphylaxis (ECF-A) are known to be released along with histamine from mast cells and basophils as a consequence of an IgE-mediated reaction. SRS-A, in contrast to histamine, causes a slow prolonged contraction of guinea pig ileum and human bronchial smooth muscle which is not antagonized by antihistamines. The role of eosinophils in these reactions has yet to be explained satisfactorily.

1.8.3. Parasitic Infections

Immunological mechanisms involving histamine, mast cells and basophils, and IgE antibodies have been implicated in resistance to infection by certain parasitic worms (nematodes, cestodes, and trematodes), among which may be mentioned *Ascaris, Trichinella,* and *Schistosoma*. The formation of IgE antibodies is a general phenomenon which is part of the immune response in helminth-infected animals. These antibodies are readily detected by direct skin test with crude worm antigens, and their presence in the serum of an infected individual can be detected by passive transfer test. Marked elevation of total serum IgE level occurs in infected humans. Still, the role of IgE antibodies in resistance to these worms has not yet been determined, as the mechanisms of resistance are not completely understood.

Some evidence concerning the possible role of histamine in the inflammatory reaction to parasitic worms has been provided by studies of *Nippostrongylus brasiliensis* infection in the rat (Murray *et al.*, 1971). IgE and IgG antibodies can be detected in the serum within 10 days after a primary infection with this intestinal helminth; beginning at about 14 days, most of the worms are rapidly expelled from the intestines, the so-called self-cure reaction. Beginning several days before worm expulsion, there is a marked increase in the mucosal content of mast cells and histamine, and the mast cells are sensitized by worm-specific IgE antibody. During the rapid phase of worm expulsion, many of the mucosal mast cells degranulate, presumably as a consequence of reaction with antigens secreted by the nearby worms. Degranulation is accompanied by a marked decline of intestinal histamine content; increased permeability of the intestinal mucosa has also been demonstrated. It has been suggested that histamine and other biogenic amines released from the mucosal mast cells by the IgE-mediated reaction are responsible for the altered mucosal permeability. It was further hypothesized that this change enhances the transfer of antiworm antibodies of the IgG class into the intestinal lumen where they can damage the worms. Expulsion of worms may also require sensitized lymphocytes (Kelly and Dineen, 1972). Thus studies with this model have suggested an important role for histamine in the inflammatory reaction associated with this infection, although it is not agreed that amine release is involved in worm expulsion (Dineen et al., 1973). Therefore, a general statement about the participation of histamine, mast cells, and IgE antibodies in resistance to parasitic worms cannot be made yet.

1.8.4. Immune Complex Disease

Another inflammatory condition in which histamine appears to be involved as a chemical mediator is the so-called immune complex disease (ICD). When circulating immune complexes are deposited at multiple vascular sites, an inflammatory reaction develops; glomerulonephritis, vasculitis, and endocarditis are the common lesions of this syndrome. It has been suggested by observations of experimental ICD in rabbits that the passive deposition of immune complexes from the blood is dependent on a state of enhanced vascular permeability (Cochrane and Koffler, 1973). Acute ICD, also known as "serum sickness," is induced by a single large injection of protein antigen. As the immune response occurs, soluble circulating antigen–antibody complexes are formed. These become deposited in the glomeruli and in the walls of large arteries, where characteristic inflammatory lesions are produced. The passive deposition of these complexes is dependent on a state of enhanced vascular permeability. As noted previously, the main reservoir of histamine in the blood of rabbits is the platelets. These cells appear to be the source of the histamine that triggers increased vascular permeability; depletion of platelets reduces the deposition of immune complexes. Four different immunological reactions can lead to the release of histamine from rabbit platelets. Three of them require complement and immune complexes at equivalence or in antibody excess. The fourth requires the participation of basophils sensitized by IgE antibody and does not require complement. Observations of this reaction in vitro show platelets aggregating around basophils shortly after the addition of antigen. Recent evidence indicates that the reaction of antigen with basophils sensitized by IgE antibody results in the release of a substance called "platelet-activating factor" (PAF). This substance binds readily to platelets, neutrophils, and serum albumin. PAF induces platelets to aggregate and to secrete histamine, serotonin, and nucleotides. It is thought that this sort of reaction may occur at sites of turbulence within the vasculature. Changes in vascular permeability result from the local release of amines from platelets and lead to trapping of antigen–antibody complexes along the basement membrane. Once deposited, these complexes may lead to tissue injury by leukocyte-dependent or -independent mechanisms. This evidence is consistent with but certainly does not prove the hypothesis that these chemical mediators are involved in the pathogenesis of this inflammatory process. The involvement of histamine and serotonin from platelets in ICD in rabbits is further supported by experiments in which the deposition of complexes could be prevented by continuous treatment of the animals with both histamine and serotonin antagonists. The development of chronic immune complex–induced glomerulonephritis in rabbits was reduced by commencing continuous administration of these antagonists both before the onset of the renal lesion and after the lesion had become established (Knicker, 1972). Preliminary evidence has been obtained for the release of PAF from human basophils (Benveniste, 1974), suggesting that the above mechanism may also be involved in the pathogenesis of serum sickness in man. In a recent clinical trial, prophylactic administration of cyproheptadine, an antagonist of both histamine and serotonin, apparently reduced the incidence of acute serum sickness in patients who received a single dose of horse anti-diphtheria toxin globulin (Knicker, 1972). However, it is still too early to be certain of the relative significance of the involvement of histamine in the pathogenesis of these lesions.

1.8.5. Mast Cells and Basophils in Other Immunological Reactions

The recent studies of Dvorak (Dvorak *et al.*, 1970; Dvorak, 1971; Dvorak and Mihm, 1972) have drawn attention to the involvement of basophils and mast cells and therefore of histamine in several immunological reactions which heretofore were regarded as involving primarily lymphocytes and monocytes. In guinea pigs, a reaction which Dvorak termed "cutaneous basophil hypersensitivity" (CBH) was induced with proteins in incomplete Freund's adjuvant or in saline; this reaction is delayed in onset like classical delayed hypersensitivity and is characterized morphologically by massive infiltration of the dermis with basophilic leukocytes. Mononuclear cells and small lymphocytes are also present. Dense infiltrates of basophils have been demonstrated in guinea pigs with contact dermatitis, immunity to viruses and to ticks, allograft rejection, and tumor immunity. Similar cellular infiltrates have been observed in human allergic contact dermatitis. Also seen in these lesions are dermal edema and vascular compaction, which suggest increased vascular permeability resulting from the action of histamine and other chemical mediators, presumably released by the basophils which, however, are not degranulated.

Colvin and Dvorak (1974) reported that basophils accounted for 40% of the infiltrating granulocytes in biopsy specimens obtained from patients undergoing acute cellular rejection of human allografts. Mast cells, normally scarce in the human kidney, were increased more than tenfold above normal in the cortical interstitium and around small blood vessels in these biopsies. Dvorak believes that basophils are quickly mobilized, short-lived cells which participate in sensitized hosts in the initial response to antigen and that basophils are replaced by mast cells in more chronic processes. He hypothesized the existence of interaction between basophils or mast cells and thymus-derived lymphocytes in these immune reactions; that is, there may be synergism between immediate hypersensitivity, which is mediated by IgE antibody, and classic cell-mediated immunity. Reports that the cytolytic activity of "immune" thymus-derived lymphocytes can be suppressed by histamine (Henney *et al.*, 1972) and that this inhibition can be antagonized by burimamide (Plaut *et al.*, 1973) are consistent with the idea of modulation of leukocyte functions by histamine and other mediators released by mast cells and basophils (Bourne *et al.*, 1974). There is obviously much more to learn about the role of histamine in inflammation and in the immune response.

2. SEROTONIN

Serotonin is an endogenous biogenic amine which, like histamine, has potent effects on small blood vessels and on smooth muscles in certain mammalian species (Udenfriend and Waalkes, 1959). Like histamine, its role in inflammation still needs further definition. Its most important functions may concern the nervous system and the gastrointestinal tract.

Serotonin was first identified by Erspamer (1954) as a pharmacologically active factor from enterochromaffin cells of the intestinal tract. Chemically, it is 5-hydroxytryptamine, or 3-(2-aminoethyl)-5-indolol; its molecular weight is 176; it is soluble in water and glacial acetic acid but insoluble in absolute ethanol, ether, and chloroform. It can be assayed fluorometrically or by bioassay with rat colon or estrous rat uterus. In the latter method, serotonin is identified by showing that lysergic acid can inhibit muscle contractions induced by the test sample.

In mammalian tissues, serotonin is localized in enterochromaffin cells of the mucosal layer of the gastrointestinal tract. The gut contains about 1 μg of serotonin/g tissue; carcinoid tumors of the enterochromaffin cells may contain 1000 times this amount. Parts of the brain also contain significant amounts of serotonin; for example, the hypothalamus contains about 1 μg/g tissue. Rat, mouse, and rabbit lung are another site of serotonin storage; human and guinea pig lung do not contain serotonin. In most mammals, platelets are the reservoir of serotonin in the blood. Human blood contains about 0.1–0.2 μg/ml. Rat and mouse mast cells are rich in serotonin, whereas the mast cells of most other mammals do not contain it. Rat peritoneal mast cells contain from 0.2 to 6.0 μg of serotonin/10^6 cells; in these cells, serotonin is stored in the same cytoplasmic granules that contain histamine (Austen, 1971).

Serotonin is derived from the amino acid tryptophan by hydroxylation to 5-hydroxytryptophan, which is then decarboxylated to yield serotonin (Fig. 2). After its release, it is oxidized by monoamine oxidase to 5-hydroxyindole acetic acid, which is then excreted in the urine.

The principal pharmacological properties of serotonin are the induction of smooth muscle contraction and increased vascular permeability (Spector and Willoughby, 1968). Its effect on smooth muscle shows considerable species variation; for instance, rat smooth muscle is very sensitive to serotonin (but relatively insensitive to histamine), whereas human smooth muscle is relatively insensitive to it. Its effect on postcapillary venules closely resembles the actions of histamine; that is, gaps are produced between endothelial cells and local transudation of plasma ensues. These effects can be antagonized by dibenamine hydrochloride and lysergic acid derivatives as well as by some drugs which also antagonize histamine, e.g., cyproheptadine (Periactin).

Serotonin is released *in vitro* from rabbit platelets together with histamine by immune complexes in the presence of complement (Gocke and Osler, 1965) and by the basophil-dependent, IgE antibody–mediated, complement-independent mechanism (Cochrane and Koffler, 1973). These same biogenic amines can be released from rat peritoneal mast cells *in vitro* by a variety of agents, including IgE and IgG antibody–dependent reactions, C3a and C5a anaphylatoxins, neutrophil-derived cationic proteins, and low molecular weight

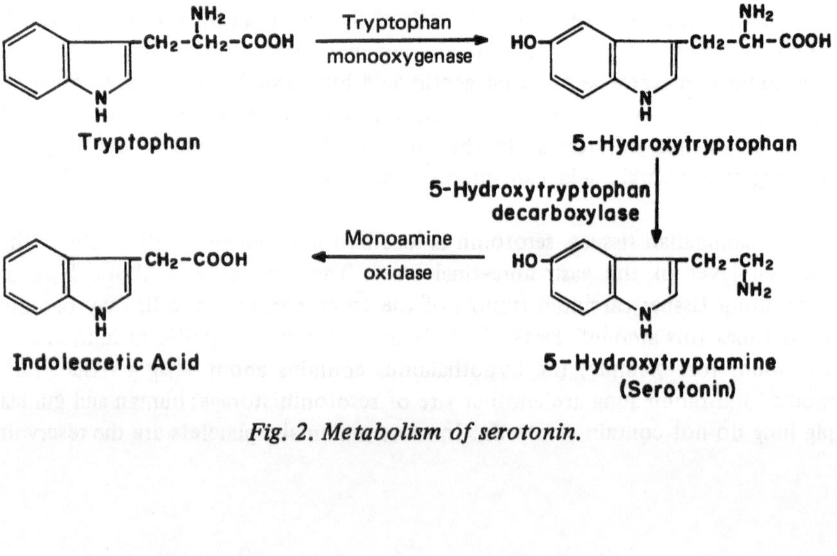

Fig. 2. Metabolism of serotonin.

substances such as compound 48/80, polymyxin B, and ATP (Morrison *et al.*, 1974). Thus it seems logical to believe that serotonin may be involved in anaphylactic reactions in the rat and mouse at least, since release of the amine can be demonstrated under appropriate conditions, since serotonin can induce changes characteristic of anaphylaxis, and since the signs of local and systemic anaphylaxis can be blocked with a serotonin antagonist in these two species. It may have little to do with anaphylactic reactions in other species. However, serotonin released from platelets may participate along with histamine in the mediation of immune complex disease in rabbits and humans (Knicker, 1972; Cochrane and Koffler, 1973). Beyond these situations, there is little direct evidence implicating serotonin as a mediator of inflammation (Spector and Willoughby, 1968). Its role in normal physiological processes is probably more important.

3. REFERENCES

Ackermann, D., 1910, Über den bacteriellen Abbau des Histidins, *Z. Physiol. Chem.* **65**:504.

Ash, A. S. F., and Schild, H. O., 1966, Receptors mediating some actions of histamine, *Brit. J. Pharmacol.* **27**:427.

Austen, K. F., 1971, Histamine and other mediators of allergic reactions, in: *Immunological Diseases*, 2nd ed. (M. Samter, ed.), pp. 332–355, Little, Brown, Boston.

Barger, J., and Dale, H. H., 1910, The presence in ergot and physiological activity of β-imidazolylethylamine, *J. Physiol. (Lond.)* **40**:XXXVIII.

Bartosch, R., Feldberg, W., and Nagel, E., 1932, Das Freiwerden eines histaminähnlichen Stoffes bei der Anaphylaxie des Meerschweinchens, *Pfluegers Arch. Ges. Physiol.* **230**:129.

Beall, G. N., and VanArsdel, P. P., Jr., 1960, Histamine metabolism in human disease, *J. Clin. Invest.* **39**:676.

Benveniste, J., 1974, Characteristics and semipurification of a platelet activating factor from human and rabbit leukocytes, *Fed. Proc.* **33**:797 (abst.).

Black, J. W., Duncan, W. A. M., Durant, C. J., Genellin, C. R., and Parsons, E. M., 1972, Definition and antagonism of histamine H_2-receptors, *Nature (Lond.)* **236**:385.

Bloch, K. J., 1973, Reaginic and other homocytotropic antibodies: Diverse immunoglobulins with common function, in: *Mechanisms in Allergy* (L. Goodfriend, A. H., Sehon, and R. P. Orange, eds.), pp. 11–32, Dekker, New York.

Bourne, H. R., Lichtenstein, L. M., Melmon, K. L., Henney, C. S., Weinstein, Y., and Shearer, G. M., 1974, Modulation of inflammation and immunity by cyclic AMP, *Science* **184**:19.

Brody, M. J., Håkanson, R., Ourman, C., and Sundler, F., 1972, An improved method for the histochemical demonstration of histamine and other compounds producing fluorophores with *o*-phthaldialdehyde, *J. Histochem Cytochem.* **29**:945.

Chakrin, L. W., Mengel, J., Young, D., Zaher, C., Krell, R. D., and Wardell, J. R., Jr., 1974, Enhancement of immediate-type hypersensitivity reactions by *N*-methyl-*N'*-(2((4-methyl-5-imidazolyl)methylthio)ethyl)thiourea, *Fed. Proc.* **33**:585 (abst.).

Cochrane, C. G., and Koffler, D., 1973, Immune complex disease in experimental animals and man, *Advan. Immunol.* 16:185.

Colvin, R. B., and Dvorak, H. F., 1974, Basophils and mast cells in renal allograft rejection, *Lancet* 1:212.

Dale, H. H., 1929, On some chemical factors in the control of circulation, Croonian lectures, II and III, *Lancet* 216:1232, 1285.

Dale, H. H., and Laidlaw, P. P., 1910, The physiological action of β-iminazolylethylamine, *J. Physiol. (Lond.)* 41:318.

Dineen, J. K., Ogilvie, B. M., and Kelly, J. D., 1973, Expulsion of *Nippostrongylus brasiliensis* from the intestine of rats, *Immunology* 24:467.

Dragstedt, C. A., and Gebauer-Fuelnegg, E., 1932, Studies in anaphylaxis: The appearance of a physiologically active substance during anaphylactic shock, *Am. J. Physiol.* 102:512.

Dvorak, H. F., 1971, Role of the basophilic leukocyte in allograft rejection, *J. Immunol.* 106:279.

Dvorak, H. F., and Mihm, M. C., Jr., 1972, Basophilic leukocytes in allergic contact dermatitis, *J. Exp. Med.* 135:235.

Dvorak, H. F., Dvorak, A. M., Simpson, B. A., Richerson, H. B., Leskowitz, S., and Karnovsky, M. J., 1970, Cutaneous basophil hypersensitivity. II. A light and electron microscopic description, *J. Exp. Med.* 132:558.

Eppinger, H. 1913, Über eine eigentumliche Hautreaktion hervogerufen durch Ergamin, *Wien. Med. Wschr.* 63:1414.

Erspamer, V., 1954, Pharmacology of indolealkylamines, *Pharmacol. Rev.* 6:425.

Gocke, D. J., and Osler, A. G., 1965, *In vitro* damage of rabbit platelets by an unrelated antigen–antibody reaction. I. General characteristics of the reaction, *J. Immunol.* 94:236.

Håkanson, R., and Liedberg, G., 1971, Evidence against histamine as final chemostimulator of gastric acid secretion, *Am. J. Physiol.* 221:641.

Henney, C. S., Bourne, H. R., and Lichtenstein, L. M., 1972, The role of cyclic 3′,5′-adenosine monophosphate in the cytolytic activity of lymphocytes, *J. Immunol.* 108:1526.

Kahlson, J., and Rosengren, E., 1971, *Biogenesis and Physiology of Histamine,* Williams and Wilkins, Baltimore.

Kelly, J. D., and Dineen, J. K., 1972, The cellular transfer of immunity to *Nippostrongylus brasiliensis* in inbred rats (Lewis strain), *Immunology* 22:199.

Knicker, W. T., 1972, Modulation of the inflammatory response *in vivo:* Prevention or amelioration of immune complex disease, in: *Inflammation: Mechanisms and Control* (I. H. Lepow and P. A. Ward, eds.), pp. 335–367, Academic Press, New York.

Levi, R., 1972, Effects of exogenous and immunologically released histamine on the isolated heart: A quantitative comparison, *J. Pharmacol.* 182:227.

Levi, R., and Lee, C.-H., 1974, Characterization of cardiac receptors by means of selective H_1- and H_2-agonists and antagonists, *Fed. Proc.* 33:585 (abst.).

Levine, R. J., 1968, Histamine and the effect of gastrin on gastric acid secretion in man, *Fed. Proc.* 27:1341.

Lewis, T., 1927, *Blood Vessels of the Human Skin and Their Responses,* Shaw, London.

Lichtenstein, L. M., 1972, Allergy, in: *Clinical Immunobiology,* Vol. 1 (F. H. Bach and R. A. Good, eds.), pp. 243–269, Academic Press, New York.

Lichtenstein, L. M., and Gillespie, E., 1973, Inhibition of histamine release by histamine controlled by H_2 receptor, *Nature (Lond.)* 244:287.

Majno, G., 1965, Ultrastructure of the vascular membrane, in: *Handbook of Physiology,* Vol. 3, Sect. 2 (J. Field, ed.), pp. 2293–2375, Williams and Wilkins, Baltimore.

May, D. C., Lyman, M., Alberto, R., and Cheng, J., 1970, Procedures for immunochemical study of histamine release from leukocytes with small volumes of blood, *J. Allergy* **46**:12.

Melmon, K. L., Bourne, H. R., Weinstein, J., and Sela, M., 1972, Receptors for histamine can be detected on the surface of selected leukocytes, *Science* **177**:707.

Morrison, D. C., Roser, J. F., Henson, P. M., and Cochrane, C. G., 1974, Activation of rat mast cells by low molecular weight stimuli, *J. Immunol.* **112**:573.

Murray, M., Jarrett, W. F. H., and Jennings, F. W., 1971, Mast cells and macromolecular leak in immunological reactions, *Immunology* **21**:17.

Plaut, M., Lichtenstein, L. M., Gillespie, E., and Henney, C. S., 1973, Studies on the mechanism of lymphocyte-mediated cytolysis. IV. Specificity of the histamine receptor on effector T cells, *J. Immunol.* **111**:389.

Portier, P., and Richet, C., 1902, De l'action anaphylactique de certains venins, *Compt. Rend. Soc. Biol.* **54**:170.

Powell, J. R., and Brody, M. J., 1974, Identification of two vascular histamine (hist) receptors in the dog, *Fed. Proc.* **33**:585 (abst.).

Riley, J. F., 1953, Histamine in tissue mast cells, *Science* **118**:332.

Rocha e Silva, M., 1955, *Histamine—Its Role in Anaphylaxis and Allergy*, Charles C Thomas, Springfield, Ill.

Rocha e Silva, M. (sub-ed.), 1966, Histamine: Its chemistry, metabolism and physiological and pharmacological actions, in: *Handbook of Experimental Pharmacology*, Vol. XVIII/1 (O. Eichler and A. Farah, eds.), Springer-Verlag, New York.

Schayer, R. W., 1965, Histamine and circulatory homeostasis, *Fed. Proc.* **24**:1295.

Selye, H., 1965, *The Mast Cells*, Butterworths, London.

Shore, P. A., Burkhalter, A., and Cohn, V. H., Jr., 1959, A method for the fluorometric assay of histamine in tissues, *J. Pharmacol. Exp. Ther.* **127**:182.

Snyder, S. H., Baldessarini, R. J., and Axelrod, J., 1966, A sensitive and specific enzymatic isotopic assay for tissue histamine, *J. Pharmacol. Exp. Ther.* **153**:544.

Spector, W. G., and Willoughby, D. A., 1968, *The Pharmacology of Inflammation*, Grune and Stratton, New York.

Taylor, K. M., and Snyder, S. H., 1972, Isotopic microassay of histamine, histidine, histidine decarboxylase, and histamine methyltransferase in brain tissue, *J. Neurochem.* **19**:1343.

Udenfriend, S., and Waalkes, T. P., 1959, On the role of serotonin in anaphylaxis, in: *Mechanisms of Hypersensitivity* (J. H. Shaffer, G. A. LoGrippo, and M. W. Chase, eds.), pp. 219–226, Little, Brown, Boston.

Uvnäs, B., 1967, Mode of binding and release of histamine in mast cell granules from the rat, *Fed. Proc.* **26**:219.

Windaus, A., and Vogt, W., 1907, Synthese des Imidazoläthylamins, *Berichte* **40**:3691.

Wolstenholme, G. E. W., and O'Connor, C. M. (eds.), 1955, *Histamine* (Ciba Foundation Symposium), Little, Brown, Boston.

Zweifach, B. W., Grant, L., and McCluskey, R. T. (eds.), 1973, *The Inflammatory Process*, 2nd ed., Academic Press, New York.

PROSTAGLANDINS

6

Robert B. Zurier

1. INTRODUCTION

In 1930, two New York City gynecologists (Kurzrok and Lieb, 1930) observed that human myometrium exhibited rhythmic contractions and relaxation when incubated with fresh human semen. Goldblatt (1933) and von Euler (1936) independently confirmed this finding and identified the active principle as an acidic lipid, which von Euler believed to be produced in the prostate gland and therefore named "prostaglandin." Eliasson (1959) later demonstrated that prostaglandin in human semen is in fact derived from seminal vesicles. Bergström and Sjövall (1957, 1960) determined that the active component was not a single substance but several closely related compounds. These investigators isolated two of the substances in crystalline form from homogenates of sheep vesicular glands and described their chemical structure (Bergström et al., 1962).

2. CHEMISTRY

The basic structure common to all prostaglandins is a prostanoic acid skeleton, a 20-carbon-atom, unsaturated, hydroxy fatty acid with a cyclo-pentane ring at C8–C12 (Fig. 1). In nature, the prostaglandins are produced

ROBERT B. ZURIER Department of Medicine, University of Connecticut School of Medicine, Farmington, Connecticut

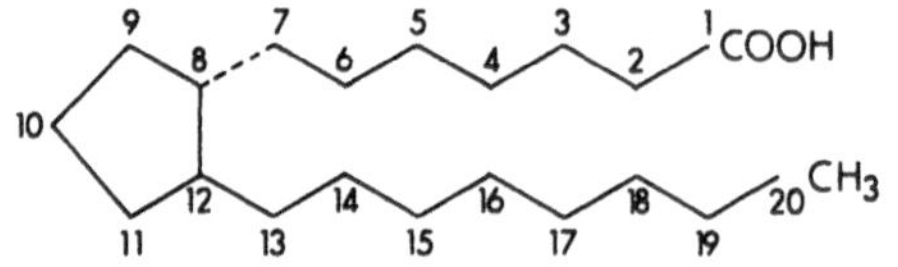

Fig. 1. Prostanoic acid. The basic structure of a fully saturated C_{20} acid, with C8–C12 closed to form a five-membered ring.

from the corresponding polyunsaturated fatty acids by a microsomal synthetase system. They are unusual among highly active biological compounds in that they lack nitrogen, in which respect they resemble the steroid hormones. The prostaglandins are grouped according to the type of chemical functionality present. Thus prostaglandins are divided into the E, F, A and B compounds by the nature of the five-membered ring functions (Fig. 2). The two main series, prostaglandins E and F (PGE, PGF), differ only in the presence of a ketone or hydroxyl function at C9. The subscript numeral after the letter indicates the degree of unsaturation in the alkyl and carboxylic side-chains. Thus whereas the numeral 1 indicates the presence of a double bond at C13–14 (PGE_1), the numeral 2 marks the presence of an additional double bond at C5–6 (PGE_2) and the numeral 3 denotes a third double bond at C17–18 (PGE_3). Substituents on the same side of the ring as the carboxyl group are in the α-position and those on the same side as the alkyl group are in the β-position: below the plane of the ring is designated α and above it β. In the presence of weak acid or alkali, the PGE compounds undergo dehydration within the ring, resulting in formation of the PGA compounds. In the presence of stronger alkali, the C10–11 double bond rearranges to the 8,12-position, and PGB compounds are formed. Thus the six naturally occurring PGE and PGF compounds are designated as primary compounds since none is a precursor of any other in this group (Fig. 3).

3. PHYSIOLOGICAL ACTIONS

The physiological role of the prostaglandins is not clear. They appear to be almost ubiquitous, having been identified in many tissues, each of which has the

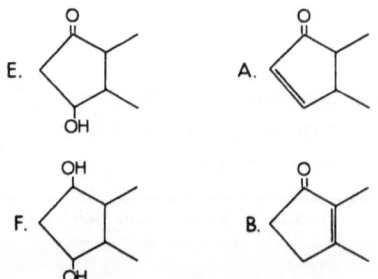

Fig. 2. Prostaglandins. Ring structures characteristic of E, F, A, and B groups.

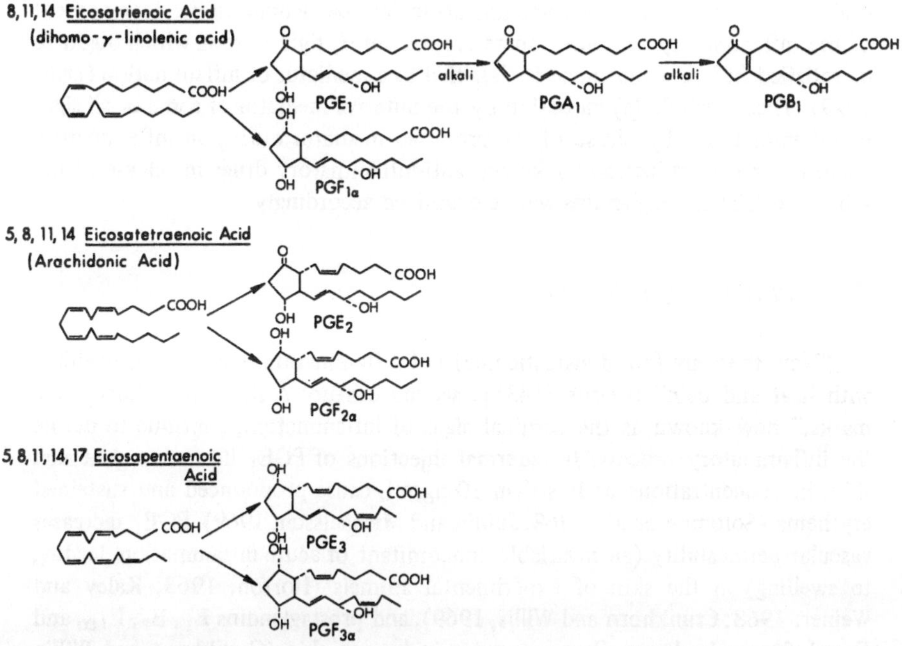

Fig. 3. Primary prostaglandins and their precursors.

capacity for synthesizing prostaglandins from essential fatty acids. It therefore seems unlikely that the prostaglandins are part of a classic endocrine–target organ system. They may, however, serve as local regulators of cell functions. The prostaglandins possess a broad spectrum of pharmacological activities (Weeks, 1972), which in several cases appear to involve changes in cyclic adenosine $3',5'$-monophosphate (cAMP) concentrations. The first of these changes to be measured was in adipose tissue (Butcher and Baird, 1968), where prostaglandins were found to decrease cAMP levels in isolated fat cells. A more usual effect of prostaglandins is to increase levels of cAMP (Hinman, 1972), by virtue of activating membrane adenyl cyclase in a manner common to the action of many hormones.

Stimulation of cells and tissues, whether by mechanical, hormonal, or neurological means, results in the increased biosynthesis of prostaglandins (Ramwell and Shaw, 1970). It has been suggested that one such stimulus is inflammation, in the course of which phospholipases are freed from the lysosomes of phagocytes (Anderson et al., 1971). These enzymes can cleave phospholipids of the cell membrane to yield arachidonic acid. This "essential" C_{20} fatty acid may in turn undergo cyclization and incorporation of molecular oxygen and be converted to prostaglandins by freely available tissue enzymes. Experimental evidence indicates that prostaglandins do in fact participate in the development of the inflammatory response. There are, however, rigid criteria which ought to be satisfied before a substance is classified as a mediator of inflammation (Dale, 1929). These include (a) induction by the putative mediator of some or all signs of inflammation, (b) release of the proposed mediator during an inflammatory reaction, and (c) reduction by known anti-inflammatory drugs in release of the substance. The prostaglandins will be examined accordingly.

3.1. Induction of Inflammation

"Now there are four diagnostic marks of inflammation: redness and swelling, with heat and pain" (Celsus [1831], second century A.D.). These "diagnostic marks," now known as the cardinal signs of inflammation, continue to define the inflammatory process. Intradermal injections of PGE_1 into normal human skin, in concentrations of less than 10 ng/ml, cause pronounced and sustained erythema (Solomon *et al.*, 1968; Juhlin and Michaelsson, 1969). PGE_1 increases vascular permeability (an invariable concomitant of acute inflammation, leading to swelling) in the skin of experimental animals (Horton, 1963; Kaley and Weiner, 1968; Crunkhorn and Willis, 1969), and prostaglandins E_1, E_2, $F_{1\alpha}$, and $F_{2\alpha}$ induce wheal and flare responses in human skin (Crunkhorn and Willis, 1971a; Søndergaard and Greaves, 1971). The permeability effects of the prostaglandins in man appear due to a direct action or the microvasculature and not to release of vasoactive substances such as histamine or serotonin.

The heat associated with inflammation is probably due in large measure to local hyperemia (Metchnikoff, 1905). There is evidence (Lewis, 1971) that prostaglandins mediate vasodilatation in a variety of tissues.

Although it has been reported that PGE and PGF compounds do not produce pain in humans when applied to blister bases (Horton, 1965) or when injected intradermally (Willis, 1971), PGE_1 and PGE_2 do irritate the mucous membranes of the eyes (Beitch and Eakins, 1969) and airways (Cuthbert, 1971). Moreover, PGE_1 (but not PGE_2) produces writhing when injected intraperitoneally in mice (Collier and Schneider, 1972). It has also been observed that the erythematous area produced by intradermal injection of PGE_1 is sensitive to touch (Solomon *et al.*, 1968; Juhlin and Michaelsson, 1969). Whereas pain is transitory when produced in man by intradermal injections of the hydroperoxide of arachidonic acid, acetylcholine, bradykinin and histamine, pain produced by PGE_1 lasts more than 2 h (Ferreira, 1972). In addition, PGE compounds increase pain sensitivity to other chemical mediators (bradykinin, histamine). The effects of PGE_1 and PGE_2 are cumulative, depending on concentration and/or time. Therefore even minute amounts of prostaglandins, if allowed to persist at the site of injury, might in time cause pain. It has been suggested that the prostaglandins might be responsible, at least in part, for the transition from an acute to a chronic inflammatory lesion. PGE_1 and $PGF_{1\alpha}$ increase collagen biosynthesis (Blumenkrantz and Søndergaard, 1972), and might therefore be expected to enhance fibroplasia in the course of persisting inflammation.

The Greek physician Galen added loss of function as the fifth cardinal sign of inflammation. PGE_1 injections elicit inflammatory edema in rat paws in a dose—response fashion (Glenn et al., 1972), and repeated injections of PGE_2 cause a persistent swelling of the paw which interferes with ambulation (Willis and Cornelson, 1973). The injection of PGE_1 or PGE_2 into knee joints of dogs results in a severe, disabling arthritis (Rosenthale et al., 1972).

An example of immunologically induced inflammation and tissue injury, the graft vs. host reaction, reportedly is enhanced in hybrid mice which receive spleen cells from PGE_1-treated donor mice (Loose and DiLuzio, 1973).

3.2. Release During Inflammation

Among the earliest studies to implicate prostaglandins in the inflammatory response were those of Ambache et al. (1965), who showed that mechanical irritation of rabbit eyes evoked release of "irin" into the anterior chamber. In other studies (Ängaard and Samuelsson, 1964; Ambache et al., 1966; Ambache and Brummer, 1968), "irin" was identified as PGE_2 and $PGF_{2\alpha}$. Instillation into rabbit eyes of these substances is associated with vasodilatation and increased capillary permeability (Bethel and Eakins, 1971). Furthermore, intradermal injections of "irin" in man produce erythrema (Ambache, 1961).

The prostaglandin-like substances associated with several experimental models of inflammation have been regarded as terminal mediators of the acute response. Carrageenan, a sulfated mucopolysaccharide derived from Irish sea moss, *Chondrus*, induces an acute inflammatory response when injected into the paw of a rat (Winter et al., 1962). Carrageenan-induced edema of the rat foot is used widely as a model of inflammation in the search for new anti-inflammatory agents. In fact, the model has been credited with forming the basis for the discovery of indomethacin. A number of substances, including histamine, 5-hydroxytryptamine (5-HT), kinins and prostaglandins, are involved in the development of carrageenan edema. There appear to be three distinct phases of mediator release: an initial simultaneous release of histamine and 5-HT, a second phase mediated by kinins, and a third phase, the mediator of which is suspected to be prostaglandins. In experiments using histamine and 5-HT antagonists, or polymonine which depletes tissue stores of both vasoactive amines, there is a marked reduction in paw edema during the first 90 min of the inflammatory response (DiRose et al., 1971), indicating that simultaneous release of histamine and 5-HT mediates the initial phase of inflammation. Treatment of rats with cellulose sulfate (CS) lowers the plasma kininogen level about 50% (DiRose and Sorrentino, 1970), and reduces the edema during 1½–2½ h after carrageenan injection. Thus kinin appears to mediate the second phase of this particular inflammatory response. Treatment of rats with polymonine (to deplete stores of histamine and 5-HT) combined with injection of CS (to reduce kininogen) leads to total suppression of carrageenan-induced edema up to 2½ h. Willis (1969a) has demonstrated the presence of prostaglandins in inflamed paws 2½–6 h after carrageenan injection, suggesting that prostaglandins mediate the later phase of this inflammatory reaction. Activation of this third phase of inflammation requires the presence of the complement system. Depletion or blockade of the complement system prevents formation of the prostaglandin-like substance. In these experiments, however, edema fluid was squeezed from the paws and it was not certain how much of the prostaglandin-like activity was due to trauma. The carrageenan air bleb was therefore developed (Willis, 1969b) as a convenient atraumatic method for obtaining inflammatory exudate free from contamination with blood: a suspension of carrageenan in saline is injected into a subcutaneous air bleb which has been raised on the back of a rat. An inflammatory reaction ensues and samples of bleb fluid are withdrawn at various time intervals. In bleb fluid, as in exudate from the inflamed paw, histamine and kinin are found shortly after carrageenan injection, whereas prostaglandins (mainly PGE_2) appear after 3 h and reach maximum concentrations at 12–24 h (Anderson et al., 1971. Moreover, carrageenan induces prostaglandin accumulation in a dose–response manner. The concentrations of PGE_2 recovered are far in excess of those necessary to produce cutaneous inflammation. Concentrations in the bleb fluid of lysosomal β-glucuronidase and PGE_2 increase in parallel during the 24 h after carrageenan injection (Anderson et al., 1971), and it has been suggested that inflammatory cells phagocytose carrageenan, consequently releasing lysosomal phospholipases which hydrolyze phospholipids of cell membranes to yield arachidonic acid (the major precursor of PGE_2). This compound is in turn presumably converted to PGE_2 by freely available enzymes (prostaglandin synthetase). Prostaglandins (mainly PGE_2) are in fact released from rabbit polymorphonuclear leukocytes (PMNs) during phagocytosis of bacteria (Higgs and Youlton, 1972) and from human PMNs during their exposure to zymosan particles (Zurier, R. B., Willis, A. L., and Tai, H. H., unpublished observations). Explants of synovium obtained at surgery from patients with rheumatoid arthritis and maintained in organ culture produce larger amounts of prostaglandin than synovium from patients with osteoarthritis (Robinson et al., 1973). PGE_1 has been shown to be chemotactic for rabbit PMNs (Kaley and Weiner, 1971), suggesting that released prostaglandins might help perpetuate the inflammatory reaction by calling forth additional leukocytes.

Human skin possesses substrates and enzymes for the formation and metabolism of prostaglandins (Änggard and Jonsson, 1972). Increased amounts (ten- to fifteenfold of PGE_2, the major prostaglandin synthesized in skin, are found during incubation of tissue at $37°C$ and after homogenization. There is evidence (Hopkin *et al.*, 1968; Änggard *et al.*, 1972) that prostaglandins are not stored within any subcellular compartment but are formed on physiological demand, probably to act close to the site of synthesis (Änggard, 1971). They may then be inactivated by the ubiquitous prostaglandin dehydrogenase before their release into the circulation. Most processes which disturb membrane function activate the hydrolysis of arachidonic acid from phospholipids (Gilmore *et al.*, 1969), the rate-limiting step in prostaglandin biosynthesis (Samuelsson, 1970). During thermal (or mechanical) injury, cell membranes would be damaged, and with an excess of arachidonic acid at the site of prostaglandin synthetase, more than usual amounts of PGE_2 could be formed. PGE_2 is released into lymph from scalded dog paws (Änggard and Jonsson, 1971). Two phases are discerned in the vascular response to a burn injury: one immediate, lasting 5–10 min, and one delayed for 30 min, then lasting several hours to days. PGE_2, formed in skin following a burn injury, may thus be a mediator in the delayed phase of the tissue response to thermal injury and could play a role in the pathophysiology of the human burn syndrome.

Prostaglandins E_1, E_2, $F_{1\alpha}$, and $F_{2\alpha}$ have been indentified in the inflamed skin of patients with allergic contact eczema (Greaves *et al.*, 1971), and prostaglandin-like substances have been recovered from areas of delayed inflammation in skin exposed to ultraviolet radiation (Greaves and Søndergaard, 1970). The presence of a potent vasoactive substance in an inflammatory reaction does not of course permit conclusions to be drawn about its importance in the pathogenesis of the lesion, but does raise a distinct possibility the substance may be a mediator of the inflammatory response.

3.3. Effects of Anti-Inflammatory Drugs

Using a cell-free enzyme system from guinea pig lung, Vane (1971) has shown a dose-related inhibition of prostaglandin synthesis by indomethacin and aspirin. Smith and Willis (1971) found that addition of indomethacin or aspirin to washed human platelets, which they had previously shown produced PGE_2 and $PGF_{2\alpha}$ when incubated with thrombin (Smith and Willis, 1970), substantially reduced prostaglandin formation in a dose-related manner. Moreover, prostaglandin production was abolished in platelets from three subjects 1 h after they ingested 10 grains of aspirin. It has further been demonstrated (Kocsis *et al.*, 1973) that the effects of ingested aspirin persist for as long as 3 days and those of indomethacin more than 6 h. Thus in both cell-free and single-cell systems, aspirin and indomethacin inhibit synthesis of prostaglandins. Indomethacin and aspirin also abolish the release of prostaglandins normally observed when a perfused dog spleen is contracted by either catecholamines or nerve stimulation (Ferreira *et al.*, 1971). Inhibition by indomethacin or aspirin of prostaglandin release has also been shown in several other biological systems (Tomlinson *et al.*, 1972; Flower *et al.*, 1972; Collier and Flower, 1971; Aiken and Vane, 1971; Bennet and Posner, 1971; Gryglewski and Vane, 1972; Raz *et al.*, 1973; Sykes and Maddox, 1972). Since tissues do not appear to store prostaglandins, release is considered equivalent to synthesis. Other nonsteroid, anti-inflammatory substances (e.g., phenylbutazone, mefanamic acid, naproxen) also inhibit prostaglandin biosynthesis (Tomlinson *et al.*, 1972; Flower *et al.*, 1972). In contrast, dexamethasone, triamcinolone acetonide, and hydrocortisone do not inhibit prostaglandin biosynthesis significantly (Flower *et al.*, 1972). However, dexamethasone is far more effective than indomethacin as an anti-inflammatory agent. Although the anti-inflammatory steroids do not appear to inhibit prostaglandin synthetase, it is possible that they act at some other point in the prostaglandin system. Vane (1972) has suggested that the steroids might interfere with replacement of the synthetase system, with the action of prostaglandins, or with transport or release of prostaglandin precursors. With regard to the mechanism whereby aspirin and indomethacin interfere with prostaglandin biosynthesis, it has been shown (Smith and Lands, 1971) that both compounds inhibit the deoxygenase of the sheep vesicular (seminal vesicle) system in a time-dependent concentration-dependent manner, irreversibly blocking the full activity of the synthetase system.

The prostaglandins then (especially PGE_2) clearly seem able to function as mediators of inflammation.

4. PROSTAGLANDINS AS POSSIBLE MODULATORS OF INFLAMMATION

Although there is strong experimental evidence that PGE_1 and PGE_2 are local mediators of inflammation, effects on mediator release which suggest *antiphlogistic* actions have also been described. Thus PGE compounds, which increase levels of cAMP in human leukocytes (Scott, 1970; Bourne *et al.*, 1971), reduce extrusion of lysosomal enzymes from viable human leukocytes *in vitro* (Weissmann *et al.*, 1971*a,b*; Zurier *et al.*, 1973*a,b*), prevent release of histamine and slow reactive substance of anaphylaxis (SRS-A) from basophils and lung fragments (Lichtenstein and DeBernardo, 1971; Orange *et al.*, 1971), and prevent lymphocyte-mediated cytotoxicity (Henney *et al.*, 1972). PGE_1 and PGE_2 also inhibit carrageenan-induced paw edema in rats (Glenn and Rohloff, 1972) and suppress adjuvant-induced arthritis (Aspinall and Cammarata, 1969; Zurier and Quagliata, 1971; Glenn and Rohloff, 1972; Zurier and Ballas, 1973; Zurier *et al.*, 1973c) and cartilage destruction in rats, while cAMP treatment suppresses acute and chronic inflammation in several experimental models (Ichikawa *et al.*, 1972). These data suggest that PGE compounds, perhaps acting via cAMP, may inhibit as well as mediate acute and chronic inflammation.

In experiments utilizing the carrageenan–air bleb technique, placement into blebs of PGE_1 or PGE_2 in pharmacological amounts reduced (in a dose–response fashion) the rate at which inflammatory cells invaded the bleb (Zurier *et al.*, 1973c). Although PGE_1 has been reported to be leukotactic (Kaley and Weiner, 1971), inhibition by PGE_1 of chemotaxis has also been observed (Rivkin and Becker, 1972). In addition, cAMP causes inhibition of guinea pig macrophage migration (Pick, 1972). The activities in the bleb of both the cytoplasmic enzyme lactate dehydrogenase (LDH) and lysosomal β-glucuronidase are reduced by local placement of PGE_1 or PGE_2. Ultrastructural studies (Zurier *et al.*, 1973c) indicate that more lysosomes remain intact after carrageenan uptake in bleb leukocytes from PGE_1-treated animals than in leukocytes from control animals. Similarly, PGE_1 reduces degranulation and lysosomal enzyme release *in vitro* when human leukocytes encounter immune complexes (Weissmann *et al.*, 1971b, 1972; Zurier *et al.*, 1973b) and after phagocytosis by human PMNs of monosodium urate crystals (Weissmann *et al.*, 1971a, 1972; Zurier *et al.*, 1973c).

Later phases of carrageenan-induced inflammation are associated with increments in the concentration of PGE_2 in the inflammatory exudate (Anderson *et al.*, 1971). It is possible that as their concentration increases to approach "pharmacological" levels locally, prostaglandins may retard inflammation. A regulatory effect of prostaglandins is not without precedent in other systems. For example, although it is known that the prostaglandins are antilipolytic (Butcher and Baird, 1968), the lipolytic hormones will *increase* prostaglandin formation in adipose tissue of certain species (Shaw and Ramwell, 1968), suggesting that the endogenous prostaglandins may serve to attenuate hormonal stimulation of lipolysis. Such effects appear to be mediated by cAMP. A similar example of autoregulation is provided by the studies of Hedqvist (1970), who has shown that PGE_1 and PGE_2 inhibit the release of noradrenaline from the spleen in response to sympathetic nerve stimulation. PGE_2 is released by the spleen when it contracts in response to nerve stimulation. Thus by a feedback mechanism the contracting smooth muscle can reduce the stimulus which is leading to the contraction. Prostaglandin release may therefore be a defense mechanism (Collier, 1971) aimed at minimizing potential injury. Pertinent to a view of prostaglandins as local regulators of the inflammatory response is the observation (Ichikawa *et al.*, 1972) that whereas large amounts of cAMP (500 mg/kg daily for 5 days) reduce the size of preformed granulomata in rats, smaller amounts of cAMP (1 or 10 mg/kg daily for 5 days) increase the size of granulomata. In addition, whereas the capacity of PGE_1 to suppress IgE-dependent antigen-induced release of histamine from human lung tissue appears due to enhancement by PGE_1 of cellular cAMP, low concentrations of PGE_1, which decrease cAMP levels, enhance histamine release (Tauber *et al.*, 1973). Treatment of rats with PGE_1 and PGE_2 also inhibits the IgE-mediated release of SRS-A in a dose—response fashion (Koopman *et al.*, 1971). Granule movement and release of lysosomal enzymes from human leukocytes are reduced by compounds such as β-adrenergic agonists and PGE_1, which serve to enhance and sustain the usual increment in cAMP production observed when leukocyte suspensions are exposed to zymosan particles (Zurier *et al.*, 1974). Although enhanced enzyme release has not been observed when cells are treated with very low concentrations of PGE_1, it is seen when cells are incubated with cyclic guanosine monophosphate (cGMP) or with cholinergic agonists which increase cellular cGMP levels. There is evidence that $PGF_{2\alpha}$ increases cGMP in leukocytes. It is therefore possible that release of chemical mediators is controlled by changes in intracellular compounds (such as cyclic nucleotides) subsequent to alterations in local prostaglandin concentrations.

The polyarthritis of adjuvant disease in the rat has been regarded as a model for tissue injury mediated by delayed hypersensitivity (Waksman *et al.*, 1960) and has been used extensively for evaluating anti-inflammatory and immunosuppressive drugs (Newbould, 1963; Winter and Nuss, 1966). It is not clear why pharmacological doses of PGE_1 and PGE_2 (doses large enough to cause transient diarrhea and somnolence in all animals treated) prevent and suppress adjuvant arthritis (Zurier and Quagliata, 1971; Glenn and Rohloff, 1972; Zurier and Ballas, 1973; Zurier *et al.*, 1973c), but a number of possibilities are suggested by their biological effects: (a) PGE_1 increases corticosteroidogenesis in rat adrenal glands (Flack *et al.*, 1969) and stimulates release of pituitary ACTH in rats (deWied *et al.*, 1969). However, treatment with PGE_1 prevents arthritis in adrenalectomized rats (Zurier *et al.*, 1973c) (Fig. 4), suggesting that suppression of adjuvant disease by PGE_1 is not mediated solely through stimulation of the pituitary and/or adrenal glands. (b) PGE compounds reduce release of lysosomal enzymes from human leukocytes when these are exposed to immune complexes and other particles (Weissmann *et al.*, 1971a,b; Zurier *et al.*, 1973a,b). Enzyme release during phagocytosis of immune complexes is thought to be important to the pathogenesis of human rheumatoid arthritis (Zvaifler, 1970; Weissmann, 1972). Thus the protective effect of PGE_1 and PGE_2 in adjuvant arthritis might be due in part to reduced lysosomal enzyme release from phagocytic inflammatory and synovial lining cells. (c) PGE_1 reduces uptake and subsequent degradation of aggregated bovine serum albumin by mouse macrophages (Weissmann *et al.*, 1970). In the rat, PGE_1 might interfere with uptake and/or "processing" of antigen. (d) Lymphocyte populations have cytolytic activity toward cells bearing antigenic determinants against which the lymphocytes have been specifically sensitized (Rosenau and Moon, 1961). Lymphocytes from rats with adjuvant

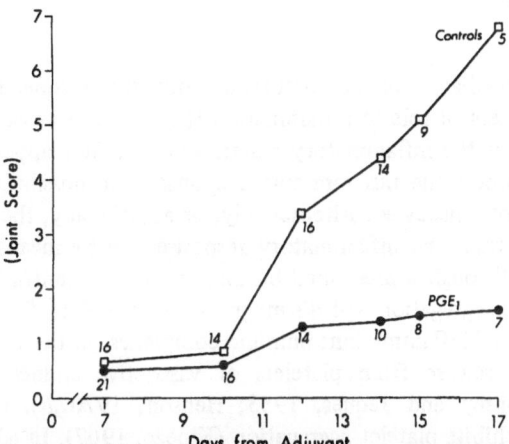

Fig. 4. Effect of PGE₁ on adjuvant arthritis in adrenalectomized rats. Each point represents the mean joint score for the number of rats noted at each point. Rats treated on days 0–15. ●, PGE_1, 300 μg s.c. twice daily; □, saline, 0.3 ml s.c. twice daily.

arthritis when injected intravenously into syngeneic rats at the time of adjuvant injection penetrate into the adjuvant-injected paw. Lymphocytes from normal rats do not enter the inflamed paw (Berney *et al.*, 1971). It appears that flow of sensitized lymphocytes through the area of high antigen concentration may help mediate the persisting inflammation. PGE_1 treatment can cause a reduction in numbers of circulating lymphocytes (Zurier *et al.*, 1973c), and lymphopenia might, in part, explain its arthritis-suppressant effect. PGE_1 *in vitro* prevents phytohemagglutinin-induced transformation of lymphocytes (Smith *et al.*, 1971), and it is conceivable that it may block lymphocyte sensitization *in vivo*. In addition, PGE_1 inhibits lymphocyte-mediated destruction of allogeneic cells *in vitro* (Henney *et al.*, 1972), suggesting an effect on T-lymphocytes. However, it is also capable of reducing the humoral antibody response (Zurier and Quagliata, 1971) and appears to prolong homograft survival through an effect on B-cells (Quagliata *et al.*, 1973). Moreover, there is experimental evidence that PGE_1 inhibits release of antibodies from splenic cells (Melmon and Bourne, 1973). Consequently, it is not clear whether PGE compounds act as "immuno-suppressants" of T- or B-cells (or both) or whether in pharmacological concentrations they inhibit release of several cell products such as mediators of inflammation and/or antibodies.

5. SUMMARY

Whether as mediators or modulators, or both, the prostaglandins appear to have a complex central role in inflammation (Fig. 5). The prostaglandins might provide balance in the inflammatory reaction in that they appear able to both mediate and suppress the inflammatory response. The possibility of feedback regulation has been discussed. Alternatively, or additionally, the prostaglandins may serve to restrain the inflammatory response, not by means of a feedback mechanism, but through a prescribed balance in local concentrations of E and F compounds. The aggregation and disintegration of platelets, for example, are a common feature of inflammation; immune complexes, in the presence of complement, induce release from platelets of vasoactive amines and lysosomal enzymes (Humphrey and Jaques, 1955; Henson, 1970a,b). PGE_2 enhances whereas PGE_1 inhibits platelet aggregation (Kloeze, 1967). In addition, $PGF_{2\alpha}$ inhibits the increases in vascular permeability induced in skin by PGE_1 and PGE_2 (Crunkhorn and Willis, 1971b). The formation of both compounds follows

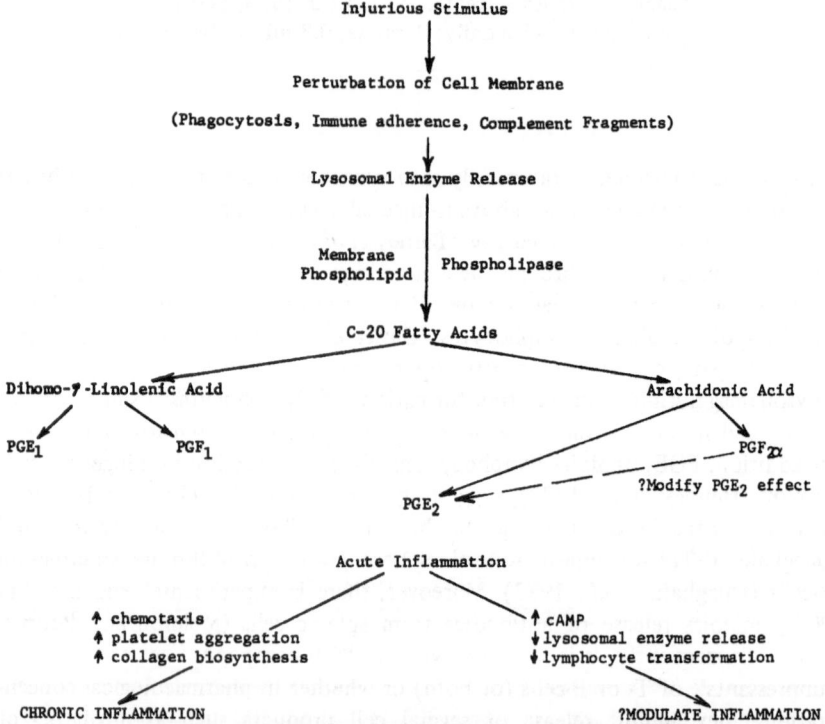

Fig. 5. Prostaglandins in the inflammatory response.

a common pathway until the final stage of biosynthesis, and there is no evidence for interconversion between E and F prostaglandins. Local control of inflammation might therefore result from the preferential biosynthesis of one or another of the prostaglandins.

6. REFERENCES

Aiken, J. W., and Vane, J. R., 1971, Blockade of angiotensin-induced prostaglandin release from dog kidney by indomethacin, *Pharmacologist* 13:293.

Ambache, N., 1961, Prolonged erythema produced by chromatographically purified irin, *J. Physiol. (Lond.)* 160:3.

Ambache, N., and Brummer, H. C., 1968, A simple chemical procedure for distinguishing E from F prostaglandins, with application to tissue extracts, *Brit. J. Pharmacol. Chemother.* 33:162.

Ambache, N., Kavanagh, L., and Whiting, J., 1965, Effect of mechanical stimulation on rabbits' eyes: Release of active substance in anterior chamber of perfusates, *J. Physiol. (Lond.)* 176:378.

Ambache, N., Brummer, H. C., Rose, J. G., and Whiting, J., 1966, Thin layer chromatography of spasmogenic unsaturated hydroxy acids from various tissues, *J. Physiol. (Lond.)* 185:77.

Anderson, A. J., Brocklehurst, W. E., and Willis, A. L., 1971, Evidence for the role of lysosomes in the formation of prostaglandins during carrageenan-induced inflammation in the rat, *Pharmacol. Res. Commun.* 3:13.

Änggard, E., 1971, Studies on the analysis and metabolism of the prostaglandins, *Ann. N.Y. Acad. Sci.* 180:200.

Änggard, E., and Jonsson, C. E., 1971, Efflux of prostaglandins in lymph from scalded tissue, *Acta Physiol. Scand.* 81:440.

Änggard, E., and Jonsson, C. E., 1972, Formation of prostaglandins in the skin following burn injury, in: *Prostaglandins in Cellular Biology* (P. W. Ramwell and B. B. Pharriss, eds.), pp. 269–292, Plenum, New York.

Änggard, E., and Samuelsson, B., 1964, Smooth muscle stimulating lipids in sheep iris: The identification of prostaglandin $F_{2\alpha}$, *Biochem. Pharmacol.* 13:281.

Änggard, E., and Samuelsson, B., 1965, Prostaglandins and related factors. XLII. Metabolism of prostaglandin E_2 in guinea pig lung, *Biochemistry* 4:1864.

Änggard, E., Green, K., and Samuelsson, B., 1965, Synthesis of tritium-labeled prostaglandin E_2 and studies on its metabolism in lung, *J. Biol. Chem.* 240:1932.

Änggard, E., Bohman, S. O., Griffin, J. E., Larsson, C., and Maunsbach, A. B., 1972, Prostaglandins in renal papilla, *Acta Physiol. Scand.* 84:231.

Aspinall, R. L., and Cammarata, P. S., 1969, Effect of prostaglandin E_2 on adjuvant arthritis, *Nature (Lond.)* 224:1320.

Beitch, B. R., and Eakins, K. E., 1969, The effects of prostaglandins on the intraocular pressure of the rabbit, *Brit. J. Pharmacol.* 37:158.

Bennet, A., and Posner, J., 1971, Studies on prostaglandin antagonists, *Brit. J. Pharmacol.* 42:584.

Bergström, S., 1967, Prostaglandins: Members of a new hormonal system, *Science* 157:382.

Bergström, S., and Sjövall, J., 1957, The isolation of prostaglandin, *Acta Chem. Scand.* 11:1086.

Bergström, S., and Sjövall, J., 1960, The isolation of prostaglandin E from sheep prostate glands, *Acta Chem. Scand.* 14:1701.

Bergström S., Ryhage, R., Samuelsson, B., and Sjövall, J., 1962, The structure of prostaglandins E_1, F_1, and F_2, *Acta Chem. Scand.* 16:501.

Berney, S., Bishko, F., and Quaglitata, F., 1971, Distribution of normal and sensitized lymphoid cells with adjuvant induced arthritis, *Arthritis Rheum.* 14:370.

Bethel, R. A., and Eakins, K. E., 1971, Antagonism by polyphloretin phosphate of the intraocular pressure rise induced by prostaglandins and formaldehyde in the rabbit eye, *Fed. Proc.* 30:626 (abst.).

Blumenkrantz, N., and Søndergaard, J., 1972, Effect of prostaglandins E_1 and $F_{1\alpha}$ on biosynthesis of collagen, *Nature New Biol.* 239:246.

Bourne, H. R., Lehrer, R. I., Cline, M. J., and Melmon, K. J., 1971, Cyclic 3'5'-adenosine monophosphate in the human leucocyte: Synthesis, degradation and effects on neutrophil candidacidal activity, *J. Clin. Invest.* 50:920.

Butcher, R. W., and Baird, C. E., 1968, Effects of prostaglandins on adenosine 3'5'-monophosphate levels in fat and other tissues, *J. Biol. Chem.* 243:1713.

Celsus, A. C., 1831, *De Medicina* (translated from L. Targa's edition by A. Smith), p. 182, E. Cox, London.

Collier, H. O. J., 1971, Prostaglandins and aspirin, *Nature (Lond.)* 232:17.

Collier, H. O. J., and Schneider, C., 1972, Nociceptive response to prostaglandins and analgesic actions of aspirin and morphine, *Nature New Biol.* 236:141.

Collier, J. G., and Flower, R. J., 1971, Effect of aspirin on human seminal prostaglandins, *Lancet* 2:852.

Crunkhorn, P., and Willis, A. L., 1969, Actions and interactions of prostaglandins administered intradermally in rat and man, *Brit. J. Pharmacol.* 36:216p.

Crunkhorn, P., and Willis, A. L., 1971a, Cutaneous reactions to intradermal prostaglandins, *Brit. J. Pharmacol.* 41:49.

Crunkhorn, P., and Willis, A. L., 1971b, Interaction between prostaglandins E and F given intradermally in the rat, *Brit. J. Pharmacol.* 41:507.

Cuthbert, M. E., 1971, Bronchodilator activity of aerosols of prostaglandins E_1 and E_2 in asthmatic subjects, *Proc. Roy. Soc. Med.* 64:15.

Dale, H. H., 1929, Some chemical factors in the control of the circulation, *Lancet* 1:1285.

deWied, D., Witter, A., Versteeg, D. H. G., and Mulder, A. H., 1969, Release of ACTH by substances of central nervous system origin, *Endocrinology* 85:561.

DiRose, M., and Sorrentino, L., 1970, Some pharmacodynamic properties of carrageenan in the rat, *Brit. J. Pharmacol.* 38:214.

DiRose, M., Giroud, J. P., and Willoughby, D. A., 1971, Studies of the mediators of the acute inflammatory response induced in rats in different sites of carrageenan and turpentine, *J. Pathol.* 104:15.

Eliasson, R., 1959, Studies on prostaglandins—Occurrence, formation and biological actions, *Acta Physiol. Scand.* 46:1 (Suppl. 158).

Ferreira, S. H., 1972, Prostaglandins, aspirin-like drugs and analgesia, *Nature New Biol.* 240:200.

Ferreira, S. H., Moncada, S., and Vane, J. R., 1971, Indomethacin and aspirin abolish prostaglandin release from the spleen, *Nature New Biol.* 231:237.

Flack, J. D., Jessup, R., and Ramwell, P. W., 1969, Prostaglandin stimulation of rat cortocosteroidogenesis, *Science* 163:691.

Flower, R., Gryglewski, R., Herbaczynska-Cedro, K., and Vane, J. R., 1972, Effects of anti-inflammatory drugs on prostaglandin biosynthesis, *Nature New Biol.* 238:104.

Gilmore, N., Vane, J. R., and Wyllie, J. H., 1969, Prostaglandin release by the spleen in response to an infusion of particles, in: *Prostaglandins, Peptides and Amines* (P. Mategazza and E. W. Horton, eds.), p. 21, Academic Press, London.

Glenn, E. M., and Rohloff, N., 1972, Antiarthritic and anti-inflammatory effects of certain prostaglandins, *Proc. Soc. Exp. Biol. Med.* 139:290.

Glenn, E. M., Bowman, B. J., and Rohloff, N. A., 1972, Pro-inflammatory effects of certain prostaglandins, in: *Prostaglandins in Cellular Biology* (P. W. Ramwell and B. B. Pharriss), pp. 329–344, Plenum, New York.

Goldblatt, M. W., 1933, A depressor substance in seminal fluid, *J. Soc. Chem. Ind.* 52:1056.

Greaves, M. W., and Søndergaard, J. S., 1970, Pharmacologic agents released in ultraviolet inflammation studied by continuous skin perfusion, *J. Invest. Dermatol.* 54:365.

Greaves, M. W., Søndergaard, J., and McDonald-Gibson, W., 1971, Recovery of prostaglandins in human cutaneous inflammation, *Brit. Med. J.* 2:258.

Gryglewski, R., and Vane, J. R., 1972, The release of prostaglandins and rabbit aorta contracting substance (RCS) from rabbit spleen and its antagonism by anti-inflammatory drugs, *Brit. J. Pharmacol.* 45:37.

Hedqvist, P., 1970, Studies on the effect of prostaglandins E_1 and E_2 on the sympathetic neuromuscular transmission in some animal tissues, *Acta Physiol. Scand.* 79:1 (Suppl. 345).

Henney, C. S., Bourne, H. R., and Lichtenstein, L. M., 1972, The role of cyclic 3'5'-adenosine monophosphate in the specific cytolytic activity of lymphocytes, *J. Immunol.* 108:1526.

Henson, P. M., 1970a, Mechanisms of release of constituents from rabbit platelets by antigen–antibody complexes and complement. I. Lytic and nonlytic reactions, *J. Immunol.* 105:476.

Henson, P. M., 1970b, Mechanisms of release of constituents from rabbit platelets by antigen–antibody complexes and complement. II. Interactions of platelets with neutrophils, *J. Immunol.* 105:490.

Higgs, G. A., and Youlten, L. J. F., 1972, Prostaglandin production by rabbit peritoneal polymorphonuclear leukocytes *in vitro*, *Brit. J. Pharmacol.* 44:330p.

Hinman, J. W., 1972, Prostaglandins, *Ann. Rev. Biochem.* 41:161.

Hopkin, J. M., Horton, E. W., and Whittaker, V. P., 1968, Prostaglandin content of particulate and supernatant fractions of rabbit brain homogenates, *Nature (Lond.)* 217:71.

Horton, E. W., 1963, Action of prostaglandin E_1 on tissues which respond to bradykinin, *Nature (Lond.)* 200:892.

Horton, E. W., 1965, Biological activities of pure prostaglandins, *Experientia* 21:113.

Humphrey, J. H., and Jaques, R., 1955, The release of histamine and 5-hydroxytryptamine (serotonin) from platelets by antigen antibody reactions *in vitro*, *J. Physiol. (Lond.)* 128:9.

Ichikawa, A., Nagasaki, M., Umezu, K., Hayashi, H., and Tomita, K., 1972, Effect of cyclic 3'5'-monophosphate on edema and granuloma induced by carrageenan, *Biochem. Pharmacol.* 21:2615.

Juhlin, L., and Michaelsson, G., 1969, Cutaneous vascular reactions to prostaglandins in healthy subjects and in patients with urticaria and atopic dermatitis, *Acta Dermatol. Venereol.* 49:251.

Kaley, G., and Weiner, R., 1968, in: *Prostaglandin Symposium of the Worcester Foundation for Experimental Biology* (P. W. Ramwell and J. E. Shaw, eds.), pp. 321–325, Interscience, New York.

Kaley, G., and Weiner, R., 1971, Effect of prostaglandin E_1 on leucocyte migration, *Nature New Biol.* 234:114.

Kloeze, J., 1967, Influence of prostaglandins on platelet adhesiveness and platelet aggregation, in: *Prostaglandins* (S. Bergström and B. Samuelsson, eds.), pp. 241–252, Almqvist and Wiksell, Stockholm.

Kocsis, J. J., Hernandovich, J., Silver, M. J., Smith, J. B., and Ingerman, C., 1973, Duration of inhibition of platelet prostaglandin formation and aggregation by ingested aspirin or indomethacin, *Prostaglandins* 3:141.

Koopman, W. J., Orange, R. P., and Austen, K. F., 1971, Prostaglandin inhibition of the immunologic release of slow reacting substance of anaphylaxis in the rat, *Proc. Soc. Exp. Biol. Med.* 137:64.

Kurzrock, R., and Lieb, C. C., 1930, Biochemical studies of human semen. II. The action of semen on the human uterus, *Proc. Soc. Exp. Biol. Med.* 28:268.

Lewis, G. P., 1971, Role of kinins and prostaglandins as mediators of functional hyperaemia, *Proc. Roy. Soc. Med.* 64:6.

Lichtenstein, L. M., and DeBernardo, R., 1971, The immediate allergic response: *In Vitro* action of cyclic AMP-active and other drugs on the two stages of histamine release, *J. Immunol.* 107:1131.

Loose, L. D., and DiLuzio, N. R., 1973, Effect of prostaglandin E_1 on cellular and humoral immune responses, *J. Res. Soc.* 13:70.

Melmon, K. J., and Bourne, H. J., 1973, Release of antibody from leukocytes *in vitro:* Control by vasoactive hormones and cyclic AMP, *J. Clin. Invest.* (in press).

Melmon, K. L., Weinstein, Y., Shearer, G. M., Bourne, H. R., and Bauminger, S., 1974, Separation of specific antibody-forming mouse cells by their adherence to insolubilized endogenous hormones, *J. Clin. Invest.* 53: 22.

Metchnikoff, E., 1905, *Immunity in Infective Diseases* (1968 reprint), Johnson Reprint Corp., New York.

Newbould, B., 1963, Chemotherapy of arthritis induced in rats by mycobacterial adjuvant, *Brit. J. Pharmacol.* 21:127.

Orange, R. P., Austen, W. G., and Austen, K. F., 1971, Immunological release of histamine and slow reacting substance of anaphylaxis from human lung: I. Modulation by agents influencing cellular levels of cyclic 3'5'-adenosine monophosphate, *J. Exp. Med.* 134: 136s.

Pick, E., 1972, Cyclic AMP affects macrophage migration, *Nature New Biol.* 238:176.

Quagliata, F., Lawrence, V. J. W., and Phillips-Quagliata, J. M., 1973, Prostaglandin E_1 as a regulator of lymphocyte function. Selective action on B lymphocytes and synergy with procarbazine in depression of immune responses, *Cell. Immunol.* 6: 457.

Ramwell, P. W., and Shaw, J., 1970, Biological significance of the prostaglandins, in: *Recent Progress in Hormone Research*, New York Academic Press Inc., Vol. 26, p. 37–41.

Raz, A., Stern, H., Kenig-Wakashal, R., 1973, Indomethacin and aspirin inhibition of prostaglandin E_2 synthesis by sheep seminal vesicle slices, *Prostaglandins* 3: 337.

Rivkin, I., and Becker, E. L., 1972, Possible implication of cyclic 3'5'-adenosine monophosphate in the chemotaxis of rabbit peritoneal PMN leukocytes, *Fed. Proc.* 31: 657.

Robinson, D. R., Smith, H., and Levine, L., 1973, Prostaglandin (PG) synthesis by human synovial cultures and its stimulation by colchicine, *Arthritis Rheum.* 16:129.

Rosenau, W., and Moon, H. D., 1961. Lysis of homologous cells by sensitized lymphocytes in tissue culture, *J. Natl. Cancer Inst.* 27:471.

Rosenthale, M. E., Dervinis, A., Kassarich, J., and Singer, S., 1972, Prostaglandins and anti-inflammatory drugs in the dog knee joint, *J. Pharm. Pharmacol* 24:89.

Samuelsson, B., 1970, Biosynthesis and metabolism of prostaglandins, in: *Proceedings of the Fourth International Congress of Pharmacology*, Vol. IV, p. 12, Schwabe, Basel-Stuttgart.

Scott, R. E., 1970, Effects of prostaglandins, epinephrine and NaF on human leucocyte, platelet and liver adenyl cyclase, *Blood* 35:514.

Shaw, J. E., and Ramwell, P. W., 1968, Release of prostaglandins from rat epididymal fat pad on nervous and hormonal stimulation, *J. Biol. Chem.* 243:1498.

Smith, J. B., and Willis, A. L., 1970, Formation and release of prostaglandins in response to thrombin, *Brit. J. Pharmacol.* 40:545p.

Smith, J. B., and Willis, A. L., 1971, Aspirin selectively inhibits prostaglandin production in human platelets, *Nature New Biol.* 231; 235.

Smith, J. W., Steiner, A. L., and Parker, C. W., 1971, Human lymphocyte metabolism. Effects of cyclic and noncyclic nucleotides or stimulation by phytohemagglutinin. *J. Clin. Invest.* 50: 442.

Smith, W. L., and Lands, W. E. M., 1971, Stimulation and blockade of prostaglandin synthesis, *J. Biol. Chem.* 246: 6700.

Solomon, L. M., Juhlin, L., and Kirschenbaum, M. B., 1968, Prostaglandin on cutaneous vasculature, *J. Invest. Dermatol.* 51:280.

Søndergaard, J., and Greaves, M. W., 1971, Prostaglandin E_1 effect on human cutaneous vasculature and skin histamine, *Br. J. Dermatol.* 84:424.

Sykes, J. A. C., and Maddox, I. S., 1972, Prostaglandin production by experimental tumours and effects of anti-inflammatory compounds, *Nature New Biol.* 237: 59.

Tauber, A. I., Kaliner, M., Stechschulte, D. J., and Austen, K. F., 1973, Immunologic release of histamine and slow reacting substances and anaphylaxis from human lung. V. Effects of prostaglandins on release of histamine, *J. Immunol.* 111: 27.

Tomlinson, R. V., Ringold, H. J., Qureshi, M. C., and Forchielli, E., 1972, Relationship between inhibition of prostaglandin synthesis and drug efficacy: Support for the current theory on mode of action of aspirin-like drugs, *Biochem. Biophys. Res. Commun.* 46:552.

Vane, J. R., 1971, Inhibition of prostaglandin synthesis as a mechanism of action for aspirin-like drugs, *Nature New Biol.* 231:232.

Vane, J. R., 1972, Prostaglandins in the inflammatory response, in: *Inflammation Mechanisms and Control (I. H. Lepow and P. A. Ward, eds.), pp. 261–279*, Academic Press, New York.

von Euler, U. S., 1936, On the specific vasodilating and plain muscle stimulating substances from accessory genital glands in man and certain animals (prostaglandin and vesiglandin), *J. Physiol. (Lond.)* 88:213.

Waksman, B. H., Pearson, C. M., and Sharp, J. T., 1960, Studies of arthritis and other lesions induced in rats by injection of mycobacterial adjuvant. II. Evidence that the disease is not a disseminated immunologic response to exogenous antigen, *J. Immunol.* 85:403.

Weeks, J. R., 1972, Prostaglandins, *Ann. Rev. Pharmacol.* 12:317.

Weissmann, G., 1972, Lysosomal mechanisms of tissue injury in arthritis, *New Engl. J. Med.* 286:141.

Weissmann, G., Dukor, P., and Sessa, G., 1970, Studies on lysosomes: Mechanisms of enzyme release from endocytic cells and a model for latency *in vitro*, in: *Immunopathology of Inflammation*, pp. 107–117, Excerpta Medica International Congress Series No. 229, Excerpta Medica, Amsterdam.

Weissmann, G., Dukor, P., and Zurier, R. B., 1971*a*, Effect of cyclic AMP on release of lysosomal enzymes from phagocytes, *Nature New Biol.* 231:131.

Weissmann, G., Zurier, R. B., Spieler, P. J., and Goldstein, I. M., 1971*b*, Mechanisms of lysosomal enzyme release from leukocytes exposed to immune complexes and other particles, *J. Exp. Med.* 134:149s.

Weissmann, G., Zurier, R. B., and Hoffstein, S., 1972, Leukocytic proteases and the immunologic release of lysosomal enzymes, *Am. J. Pathol.* **68**:539.

Willis, A. L., 1969*a*, Release of histamine, kinin and prostaglandin during carrageenan-induced inflammation in the rat, in: *Prostaglandins, Peptides and Amines* (P. Mantegazza and E. W. Horton, eds.), pp. 31–38, Academic Press, London.

Willis, A. L., 1969*b*, Parallel assay of prostaglandin-like activity in rat inflammatory exudate by means of cascade superfusion, *J. Pharm. Pharmacol.* **21**:126.

Willis, A. L., 1971, Prostaglandins: Their release and inter-relationship with biogenic amines, Ph.D. thesis, University of London.

Willis, A. L., and Cornelson, M., 1973, Repeated injection of prostaglandin E_2 in rat paws induces chronic swelling and a marked decrease in pain threshold, *Prostaglandins* **3**:353.

Winter, C. A., and Nuss, G. W., 1966, Treatment of adjuvant arthritis in rats with anti-inflammatory drugs, *Arthritis Rheum.* **9**:394.

Winter, C. A., Risley, E. A., and Nuss, G. W., 1962, Carrageenan-induced edema in the hind paw of the rat as an assay for anti-inflammatory drugs, *Proc. Soc. Exp. Biol. Med.* **111**:544.

Zvaifler, N., 1970, Further speculation on the pathogenesis of joint inflammation in rheumatoid arthritis, *Arthritis Rheum.* **13**:895.

Zurier, R. B., and Ballas, M., 1973, Prostaglandin E_1 suppression of adjuvant arthritis: Histopathology, *Arthritis Rheum* **16**:251.

Zurier, R. B., and Quagliata, F., 1971, Effect of prostaglandin E_1 on adjuvant arthritis, *Nature (Lond.)* **234**:304.

Zurier, R. B., Hoffstein, S., and Weissmann, G., 1973*a*, Cytochalasin B: Effect on lysosomal enzyme release from human leukocytes, *Proc. Natl. Acad. Sci.* **70**:844.

Zurier, R. B., Hoffstein, S., and Weissmann, G., 1973*b*, Mechanism of lysosomal enzyme release from human leucocytes. I. Effect of cyclic nucleotides and colchicine, *J. Cell Biol.* **58**:27.

Zurier, R. B., Hoffstein, S., and Weissmann, G., 1973*c*, Suppression of acute and chronic inflammation in adrenalectomized rats by pharmacologic amounts of prostaglandins, *Arthritis Rheum* **16**:606.

Zurier, R. B., Weissmann, G., Hoffstein, S., Kammerman, S., and Tai, H.-H., 1974, Mechanisms of lysosomal enzyme release from human leucocytes. II. Effects of cyclic adenosine monophosphate and cyclic guanosine monophosphate, autonomic agonists and agents which affect microtubule function, *J. Clin. Invest.* **53**: 297.

SLOW REACTING SUBSTANCES

7

Daniel J. Stechschulte

1. INTRODUCTION

The *in vitro* stimulation of smooth muscle preparations has been utilized to identify and initially characterize biologically active substances since the early work on the action of β-imidazolylethylamine (Dale and Laidlaw, 1910). The term "slow reacting substance" was introduced by Feldberg and Kellaway (1938) to describe the *in vitro* smooth muscle activity of material obtained during perfusion of guinea pig lung with cobra venom. Anaphylactic shock of the same tissue (Kellaway and Trethewie, 1940) produced a material with similar smooth muscle activity. In addition, the perfusion of cat paw with a condensation product of *p*-methoxyphenethylmethylamine and formaldehyde (compound 48/80) resulted in the release of a smooth muscle stimulating principle (Paton, 1951; Chakravarty *et al.*, 1959). These three slow reacting substances (SRSs) are generated by unique methods but have a common activity on the guinea pig ileum (Vogt, 1969). The physicochemical characterization of the SRSs, although not complete, has demonstrated both common and distinct properties. Additional naturally occurring substances with smooth muscle activity similar to that of the SRSs include substance P (von Euler and Gaddum, 1931), which is extractable from nervous and intestinal tissue (Lembeck and Zetler, 1971) and is now identified as an undecapeptide of 1340 mol wt (Chang and Leeman,

DANIEL J. STECHSCHULTE Department of Medicine, University of Kansas Medical Center, Kansas City, Kansas

1970), the prostaglandins and their precursors, and Darmstoff and other lipid-soluble acids (Vogt, 1958). These compounds are of biological interest and have a possible relationship to the SRSs but will not be reviewed in this Chapter.

The material generated from lung tissue and egg yolk by cobra venom phospholipase A with characteristic activity on the guinea pig ileum has been designated "SRS-C" to identify the slow reacting substances derived with cobra venom (Vogt, 1958). This term is applied to compounds with different physico-chemical properties and includes oxidation products of unsaturated fatty acids such as hydroperoxides plus prostaglandins (Vogt, 1957). Prostaglandin syn-thetase has not been demonstrated in venom, but this enzyme does exist in most tissues including the lung (Änggard and Samuelsson, 1965). Thus venom-induced release of prostaglandin F from guinea pig lung (Vogt *et al.*, 1969) is assumed to be a two-step reaction—phospholipase A activated release of prostaglandin precursors and subsequent conversion of these precursors to prostaglandin by tissue synthe-tase. Since the prostaglandins are a major component of SRS-C activity and are considered elsewhere (Chapter 6), SRS-C will not be discussed in further detail.

Slow reacting substance of anaphylaxis (SRS-A), generated from tissue by an anaphylactic reaction, was first identified as being functionally distinct from histamine by the use of histamine antagonists (Brocklehurst, 1953, 1960). Later studies described unique physicochemical properties of this substance (Chak-ravarty, 1960; Brocklehurst, 1962; Orange and Austen, 1969a; Orange et al., 1973) and clearly differentiated it from prostaglandins and other materials known to be active on smooth muscle. The perfusion fluids obtained by antigen challenge of guinea pig lung (Piper and Vane, 1969) or by 48/80 challenge of cat paw (Änggard et al., 1963) both contain prostaglandin plus SRS-A or SRS, respectively. The relationship of SRS-A to the material released by compound 48/80 from cat paw, guinea pig lung, and rat mast cells (Änggard et al., 1963) termed "slow reacting substance" (SRS) is not clear. This review will deal with these two slow reacting substances which have a common activity on smooth muscle, unique methods of generation, and many identical properties. Final determination of the chemical structures of these biologically active compounds will be necessary for a definitive comparison and assignment of terminology which is more than descriptive. At the present time, it seems advisable to retain the terms "SRS-A" and "SRS" to indicate that molecules with indistinguishable currently recognized physicochemical and biological properties are generated by unique methods.

2. SLOW REACTING SUBSTANCE (SRS)

Lipid-soluble smooth muscle stimulating materials are released from several tissues following contact with 48/80 (Änggard et al., 1963). The cat paw is a rich source of one such substance, termed "SRS," and is routinely used for its production. The *in vitro* release of SRS from cat paw by the intra-arterial injection of 48/80 at concentrations ranging from 0.001 to 25 μg/ml is optimum at a temperature of 22°C (Strandberg, 1971*a*) and requires calcium ion for maximum yield (Chakravarty *et al.*, 1959; Strandberg, 1971*b*). The release reaction is inhibited by anoxia and the absence of glucose and *N*-ethylmaleimide (Strandberg, 1971*a*). Histamine, also released by 48/80, precedes the release of SRS.

Purification of SRS (Chakravarty *et al.*, 1959; Strandberg and Uvnäs, 1971) by ethanol and ether extraction and subsequent chromatography on silicic acid demonstrated a biologically active molecule that elutes from silicic acid with a methanol–chloroform solvent (3:7 to 1:1 vol/vol). This purified material is dialyzable, indicating a low molecular weight, is labile in an acid medium, and is resistant to the enzymatic action of 15-hydroxyprostaglandin dehydrogenase (Strandberg and Uvnäs, 1971). Because of inactivation of SRS after treatment with (a) *N*,*N*'-carbo-di-*p*-tolylimide, which breaks down carboxylic acid, (b) phenyl isocyanate, which reacts with free alcoholic or phenolic hydroxyl groups, (c) acetic anhydride, which acetylates the molecule, and (d) iodine monobromide, which interacts with unsaturated double bonds, SRS was characterized by Strandberg and Uvnäs (1971) as a carboxylic acid with hydroxyl groups and one or more double bonds. The authors describe four biological activities for SRS—selective stimulation of isolated guinea pig ileum and human bronchial smooth muscle, with activity detectable at the 1 ng/ml level; increased bronchial resistance in guinea pigs studied by the Konzett–Rössler (1940) technique; increased vascular permeability in guinea pig skin with 25–100 units/site; and an increase in the blood flow in the cat hind limb without influencing systemic blood pressure. Although SRS-A has not been tested for activity in the cat hind limb, the other biological activities are identical for SRS and SRS-A. In addition, the purification techniques for SRS-A (Orange *et al.*, 1973) are similar to the techniques described by Strandberg and Uvnäs (1971). These molecules also have similar chemical characteristics. Further studies are required to determine if these "slow reacting substances" are identical molecules generated by different mechanisms.

3. SLOW REACTING SUBSTANCE OF ANAPHYLAXIS (SRS-A)

The smooth muscle contracting activity present in the effluent collected after *in vitro* antigen challenge of sensitized guinea pig lung tissue (Kellaway and Trethewie, 1940) has been subjected to extensive investigations in a number of laboratories. The term "slow reacting substance of anaphylaxis" (SRS-A) was introduced by Brocklehurst (1960) to identify immunologically generated material with characteristic pharmacological activity on smooth muscle. This designation has been extended to include a suffix superscript for the species of origin, e.g., SRS-A[rat] (Orange and Austen, 1969a). The recent demonstration that SRS-A can be released from human leukocytes (SRS-A[leuk]) has prompted the use of a superscript to identify the source of SRS-A in a given species (Grant and Lichtenstein, 1974). However, the initial characterization of SRS-A obtained from different species demonstrated identical properties (Orange et al., 1973), and if future studies demonstrate the identical chemical structure for SRS-A obtained from cells and/or tissue of all species the use of this terminology will no longer be necessary.

3.1. Pharmacological Properties

Although the chemical nature of SRS-A has not been determined, purification of the molecule has led to the description of many of its properties. The contraction of the guinea pig ileum in a standard bioassay resulted in the original detection of SRS-A (Kellaway and Trethewie, 1940). Since that time, this bioassay has been the accepted means for identification and quantitation of this substance. A pharmacological antagonist of histamine did not block the activity of SRS-A on smooth muscle (Brocklehurst, 1953, 1960). This was the first evidence that SRS-A was functionally distinct from histamine, which was known to exist in the effluent containing SRS-A. Routinely, SRS-A is assayed on a portion of guinea pig terminal ileum suspended in oxygenated Tyrode's solution at $37°C$ (Chakravarty, 1959a; Brocklehurst, 1962). The tissue is connected to a recording apparatus which responds to a change in the length of the muscle strip. After quantitated histamine contractions are established in the presence of atropine at 10^{-6} M concentration, mepyramine maleate (10^{-6} M) is added to the Tyrode's solution to abolish the histamine contractions. The addition of SRS-A to the assay bath produces a slow prolonged contraction of the ileum which reaches a plateau within 1–3 min (Orange and Austen, 1969a). The latent period prior to the onset of contraction is a function of the concentration of SRS-A added (Brocklehurst, 1963). Repeated washing of the ileum allows it to relax to its baseline length. The height of each contraction is related to the quantity of SRS-A added. A unit of SRS-A is an arbitrary designation relating to a reference sample for each laboratory (Chakravarty, 1959a; Brocklehurst, 1960) or is that concentration of SRS-A which produces a contraction on the guinea pig ileum equal in amplitude to that produced by 5 ng of histamine base (Stechschulte et al., 1967; Orange and Austen, 1974). SRS-A activity is detectable in nanogram quantities (Orange et al., 1973), and therefore 1 unit represents 1 ng or less on a weight basis.

3.1.1. Activity on Smooth Muscle

Relatively few smooth muscle preparations respond to SRS-A (Brocklehurst, 1962; Chakravarty, 1959b; Orange and Austen, 1969a), and this observation, plus the availability of selective pharmacological antagonists, permits the assessment of this molecule in a mixture of other smooth muscle stimulators. In addition to guinea pig ileum SRS-A produces a prolonged contraction on rabbit jejunum and duodenum, fowl rectal cecum and human bronchioles. Of interest is the lack of SRS-A activity on the gerbil colon, which is very sensitive to prostaglandins (Ambache, 1966), and the estrous rat uterus, which is sensitive to serotonin and bradykinin (Brocklehurst and Mawer, 1966). Brocklehurst (1962) has reported that SRS-A^{gp} is inactive on the trachea and bronchioles of the guinea pig, cat, rabbit, dog, and monkey. SRS-A is released from monkey (Ishizaka et al., 1971) and guinea pig lung tissue but apparently is not a potent in vitro stimulator of the smooth muscle of the trachea and bronchioles in these species. Using a slightly different preparation of SRS-A, Berry and Collier (1964) demonstrated in vitro constrictor activity on guinea pig bronchiole smooth muscle. Techniques for preparing highly purified SRS-A (Orange et al., 1973) are now available, and the determination of the smooth muscle profile of activity of SRS-A on homologous tissues is indicated.

3.1.2. Effect on Vascular Permeability

The evidence that SRS-A alters vascular permeability is based on the results of direct and indirect studies. Although quantitation is not precise and the preparations injected intradermally are not free of contamination, an increase in vascular permeability was observed in guinea pig and monkey epithelium with 25–50 units of SRS-A per site (Orange et al., 1969b; Orange and Austen, 1969b). Rat cutaneous vascular permeability was minimally altered with up to 125 units/site. Indirect evidence that SRS-A is active in rat skin is based on the observation that rat IgGa antibody prepares the rat peritoneal cavity for the release of vasoactive amines and SRS-A (Stechschulte et al., 1967; Morse et al., 1968). Diethylcarbamazine inhibits the release of SRS-A in the peritoneal cavity (Orange et al., 1968). In addition to preparing the peritoneal cavity for the release of mediators, IgGa antibody induces a short-latent-period homologous PCA reaction (Stechschulte et al., 1970a) which is not completely inhibited when rats are pretreated with histamine and serotonin antagonists. However, when diethylcarbamazine is added to the pretreatment regimen, complete inhibition of the PCA reaction occurs (Orange and Austen, 1969b). Final evaluation of the effect of SRS-A on vascular permeability in selected species will require a chemically pure preparation in sufficient quantity to allow a dose response over a wide range of concentrations in combination with other known mediators so that direct and synergistic activity of SRS-A can be observed.

3.1.3. Effect on Respiratory Mechanics

Only preliminary data exist on the effect of SRS-A on respiratory mechanics in man. Partially purified SRS-A of guinea pig origin in an undetermined amount given by closed circuit spirometry to four asthmatic patients produced from 10 to 28% reduction in vital capacity (Herxheimer and Stresemann, 1963). Normal individuals given 2 times this amount of SRS-A had no reduction in vital capacity. These observations are consistent with the recognized increased responsiveness of asthmatic respiratory tissue to a variety of stimuli (Curry and Lowell, 1948), but because of the lack of quantitative data relating to the units of SRS-A administered to normal individuals it cannot be concluded that SRS-A is inactive *in vivo* on normal bronchial smooth muscle.

Two experimental models in the guinea pig have been utilized to study the effects on pulmonary dynamics of intravenously (i.v.) administered SRS-A. Anesthetized normal guinea pigs prepared by the method of Konzett and Rössler (1940) demonstrate a marked increase in the resistance of the lungs to inflation following the i.v. injection with 40–160 units of charcoal-purified SRS-A[gp] (Berry *et al.*, 1963). The increased pulmonary impedance is not under the control of the sympathetic or parasympathetic nervous system. The model of Amdur and Mead (1958) utilizes unanesthetized guinea pigs in a body box and measures pulmonary compliance and resistance separately. The effects of i.v. SRS-A at doses of 500–10,000 units/kg in this system are an approximate 50% decrease in average pulmonary compliance and only modest increases in pulmonary resistance (Drazen and Austen, 1974). The effects are not mimicked by histamine, bradykinin, and prostaglandin $F_{2\alpha}$ in this system and therefore indicate a selective action for SRS-A. The results of both the aerosol administration of SRS-A to man and the i.v. administration of SRS-A to the guinea pig clearly demonstrate an *in vivo* biological activity for this compound. It is assumed that the action of administered SRS-A is in some way comparable to the effects mediated by the *in vivo* release of this substance.

3.2. Physicochemical Properties

The reliability of the bioassay for the detection of SRS-A has permitted investigators in several laboratories (Chakravarty, 1959*b*; Brocklehurst, 1962; Änggard *et al.*, 1963; Orange and Austen, 1969*a*; Orange *et al.*, 1973) to identify many of the physical and chemical properties of the molecule and/or molecules that possess this biological activity. The present evidence indicates that SRS-A from the rat, guinea pig, monkey, and human sources are similar (Orange and Austen, 1971).

3.2.1. Solubility Characteristics

The first descriptions of SRS-A activity (Kellaway and Trethewie, 1940; Brocklehurst, 1953) in an aqueous buffer indicated that this molecule was water soluble. Subsequent studies confirmed this characteristic and also demonstrated solubility in 80% ethanol, 20% pyridine, *n*-propanol, dilute ammonia, and water-saturated butanol, partial solubility in methyl alcohol, and insolubility in butanol and acetone (Chakravarty, 1960; Brocklehurst, 1962). At an acid pH, SRS-A will partition into ether; as the pH is raised to 7.0 and above, SRS-A will shift to the aqueous phase (Chakravarty, 1960; Änggard *et al.*, 1963). Ethanol-extracted SRS-A is soluble in theoretical upper phase and unlike most neutral lipids and phospholipid is not extractable with theoretical lower phase (Orange and Austen, 1969*a*).

3.2.2. Resistance to Enzymatic Destruction

The activity of SRS-A is resistant to proteolytic enzymes such as trypsin, chymotrypsin, pepsin, and activated papain (Brocklehurst, 1962); peptidases and phospholipases A, B, C, and D (Änggard *et al.*, 1963); and pronase and neuraminidase (Orange and Austen, 1969*a*; Orange *et al.*, 1973). These data indicate that SRS-A activity is not dependent on protein, peptide, phospholipid, or sialic acid structures but unfortunately do not offer positive clues as to the chemical nature of SRS-A.

3.2.3. Electrophoretic Mobility

Electrophoresis in a sucrose–water density gradient resulted in the anodal migration of SRS-A at pH 8.0 (Charlwood and Gordon, 1958). This supports the argument that SRS-A is acidic in nature. That SRS-A is acidic is confirmed by high-voltage electrophoresis of this molecule on paper at acid and alkaline pH and by the demonstration that SRS-A has an isoelectric point between pH 4.3 and 5.2, with peak activity at pH 4.7 (Orange *et al.*, 1973). Unfortunately, electrophoresis of SRS-A in any supporting medium has been associated with significant loss of biological activity, and therefore this has not been a successful technique for purification of SRS-A (Orange and Austen, 1969*a*).

3.2.4. Adsorptive Properties

The significance of the adsorptive characteristics of SRS-A is not known; however, it is possible that the *in vivo* biological activity of this molecule is modulated by attachment to various serum and tissue substances. The SRS-A[rat] activity on the guinea pig ileum, apparently lost following incubation in 50% normal rat serum at 37°C, is recoverable when the serum proteins are precipitated with 80% ethanol (Orange and Austen, 1969*a*). The pseudoglobulin fraction of serum is most active in binding SRS-A. The treatment of SRS-A in guinea pig lung perfusate with proteolytic enzymes or 80% ethanol permits this mediator to cross a dialysis membrane (Brocklehurst, 1962). Initial estimates of the molecular weight of this molecule were higher than the currently accepted molecular weight of approximately 400 (Orange *et al.*, 1973), presumably on the basis of SRS-A adsorption to other molecules. Attachment and subsequent elution of SRS-A from activated charcoal (Brocklehurst, 1962) or Amberlite (Orange *et al.*, 1973) have been utilized for purification and concentration of this material.

3.2.5. Chromatographic Purification

The use of chromatographic techniques has contributed information relative to the physicochemical properties of SRS-A and has provided an important means of purification of this mediator. Chromatography on paper was first employed by Chakravarty (1959*b*) using *n*-propanol–ammonia–water (6:3:1 vol/vol) as the development solvent in a nitrogen atmosphere. The R_f value for SRS-A was reported as 0.6–0.7. The active spot did not stain for phosphorus but following acid hydrolysis yielded a positive ninhydrin reaction. A similar R_f value was obtained by Orange *et al.* (1969*a*) using "basic" silica gel G for thin-layer chromatography. The active spot was free of sialic acid, had a negligible phosphorus content, and was separate from glucose (Orange and Austen, 1969*a*). Silicic acid chromatography of SRS-A by Änggard *et al.* (1963) and Orange *et al.* (1973) using different solvent systems resulted in significant purification. The molecular weight of 400 for SRS-A was determined by Sephadex LH20 gel filtration of a silicic acid purified preparation (Orange *et al.*, 1973). Ion exchange chromatography has not been useful because of the inability to recover SRS-A activity after subjection to this technique (Cirstea *et al.*, 1967).

3.3. In Vitro Production

The *in vitro* production of SRS-A in guinea pig lung tissue (Chakravarty and Uvnäs, 1959; Brocklehurst, 1960; Austen and Brocklehurst, 1961; Stechschulte *et al.*, 1967) and in human lung tissue (Brocklehurst, 1960; Sheard *et al.*, 1967; Parish, 1967; Orange and Austen, 1971) permitted the identification of the participating antibody, led to speculation about the cell source of this mediator, and provided much information concerning the mechanism of its release.

3.3.1. Guinea Pig Lung

Guinea pig lung tissue has provided a reliable *in vitro* source of SRS-A since the observation of Kellaway and Trethewie (1940). The studies in which this mediator is released from actively sensitized lung failed to identify the antibody responsible for preparing the tissue for antigen-induced release of SRS-A. The recognition in the guinea pig of two 7S antibodies with distinctly different biological activities (Ovary *et al.*, 1963) led to the demonstration that the electrophoretically fast, non-complement-fixing 7S IgG1 antibody sensitizes guinea pig lung fragments for the release of both histamine and SRS-A (Stech-schulte *et al.*, 1967). SRS-A is not detectable in tissue prior to antigen challenge, in contrast to histamine which is stored in the active form (Chakravarty and Uvnäs, 1959; Brocklehurst, 1960). The similar time course of release for histamine and SRS-A, the inhibition of release at temperatures of 17–32°C and at pH values below 7.0, and the requirement of oxygen and calcium ions for release of both mediators prompted Chakravarty and Uvnäs (1959) to speculate that both histamine and SRS-A were released from the same cell source. These findings, plus the observation that the release of histamine and SRS-A was related to a decrease in the number of tissue mast cells, led to the suggestion that the mast cell was the source of SRS-A (Boreus and Chakravarty, 1960). Brocklehurst (1960) observed a slightly different time course of release for histamine and SRS-A and an inconstant relationship between the quantities of histamine and SRS-A released, and did not conclude that the mast cell was the source of SRS-A. The recent description of techniques for obtaining suspensions of viable cells from rabbit lung (Clements *et al.*, 1972) should be applicable to guinea pig lung and provide the opportunity to definitively identify the cell or substrate from which SRS-A is derived.

Enhancement of both histamine and SRS-A release from chopped guinea pig lung (Austen and Brocklehurst, 1961) was observed in the presence of dibasic aliphatic acids such as succinic and maleic. Monobasic fatty acids inhibit the release of these mediators. The mechanisms by which these compounds enhance or inhibit SRS-A release have not been defined. Prolonged incubation of the tissue with these agents is not required for their effect. This indicates that the cell membrane may be the site of their action.

The pharmacological control of SRS-A release from guinea pig lung is not well studied. The first evidence for epinephrine inhibition or antigen-induced histamine release was reported with the guinea pig lung model (Schild, 1936), and extensive studies in several laboratories have defined the mechanisms of histamine release (Mongar and Schild, 1962). It is likely that the formation and release mechanisms for SRS-A in guinea pig lung are similar to those described for histamine release. The above data indicate that SRS-A is present in an inactive form associated with an unidentified guinea pig lung cell (possibly the mast cell) prior to antigen challenge. The release of SRS-A requires optimum temperature and pH and an adequate concentration of calcium ions and oxygen. The antigen-activated step leading to the release of SRS-A can be inhibited by a variety of enzymes, by the presence of diisopropyl fluorophosphate (DFP) at the time of antigen challenge (Becker, 1959), and by monobasic fatty acids. Enhancement of SRS-A release with aliphatic four-carbon dibasic acids further defines the events involved in the production and release of this mediator initiated by an antigen–antibody reaction.

3.3.2. Human Lung

Human lung tissue was identified as a source of SRS-A by the observation of Brocklehurst (1960). The exposure of human asthmatic lung tissue *in vitro* to appropriate antigens resulted in the release of both histamine and SRS-A. The subsequent observation (Parish, 1967; Sheard *et al.*, 1967) that human lung tissue could be passively sensitized *in vitro* with atopic serum for antigen-induced release of these mediators led to studies which specifically identified IgE antibody in atopic serum as the responsible immunoglobulin for preparing lung tissue for the release of SRS-A as well as other mediators (Orange *et al.*, 1971; Kay and Austen, 1971). The short-term sensitizing IgG antibody (Parish, 1973) has not been examined for its capacity to prepare human lung tissue for the release of mediators. In general, the release of SRS-A from human lung parallels the release of histamine. However, recent studies (Orange, 1974) demonstrate that control of histamine release can be dissociated from the control of SRS-A release by antigen challenge in the presence of cytochalasins A and B. As in guinea pig lung, the cell source of SRS-A from human lung has not been identified. However, IgE antibody is known to attach to primate tissue mast cells (Ishizaka *et al.*, 1972), and this indicates that the release reaction is initiated at the mast cell membrane level. These observations, plus the finding that human lung cell suspensions rich in mast cells release both histamine and SRS-A when challenged with monospecific antisera against IgE (Lewis *et al.*, 1974) and the similar observation with suspensions of primate lung cells (Ishizaka *et al.*, 1972), clearly focus attention on the tissue mast cell.

The metabolic requirements for the release of SRS-A from human lung tissue (Orange *et al.*, 1971) include an intact glycolytic pathway, as demonstrated by inhibition with the addition of 2-deoxyglucose to glucose-free Tyrode's solution and inhibition by the addition of iodoacetic acid to the buffer solution. The iodoacetic acid inhibition at the 3-phosphoglyceraldehyde dehydrogenase step is prevented by the addition of pyruvate, thus bypassing this block. In addition, the antigen-induced release of both histamine and SRS-A from human lung tissue is inhibited in the presence of diisopropyl fluorophosphate (Orange *et al.*, 1971). In contrast to the release of histamine, the release of SRS-A is partially inhibited by preincubation of tissue with DFP. This suggests that the esterase involved in SRS-A release is already in a DFP-sensitive form or that residual DFP has remained in the tissue even after washing. As in other tissues, calcium is required for the release of both histamine and SRS-A (Austen, 1973). Dibasic acids such as succinic and maleic enhance the release of both mediators from human lung (Orange *et al.*, 1971). Thus it appears that the formation and release of SRS-A from human lung are initiated by an IgE antibody–antigen interaction at the surface of the mast cell. The release process is characterized by a series of events which are under specific biochemical controls. Most studies are compatible with the view that the secretory processes for both mediators are identical. Preliminary data suggest that the formation of SRS-A may be a unique process.

The pharmacological control of SRS-A release from human lung tissue has been extensively studied. Disodium cromoglycate at concentrations of 10–15 μg/ml inhibits the antigen-induced release of both histamine and SRS-A from human lung (Sheard and Blair, 1970; Assem and Mongar, 1970); however, at concentrations of 50 and 100 μg/ml no inhibition is observed (Orange and Austen, 1971). Diethylcarbamazine, initially observed to inhibit the release of SRS-A in the rat peritoneal cavity (Orange et al., 1968), also inhibits the release of histamine and SRS-A from human lung (Orange and Austen, 1971). The mechanism of action of both disodium cromoglycate and diethylcarbamazine in inhibiting mediator release requires further definition.

Data obtained with human lung fragments indicate that the antigen-induced release of histamine and SRS-A is modulated by α- and β-adrenergic as well as cholinergic stimulation (Kaliner et al., 1972). Lung tissue incubated with β-adrenergic agents reflects an increase in the cellular level of cyclic adenosine 3′,5′-monophosphate (cAMP) associated with inhibition of antigen-induced mediator release (Orange et al., 1971). α-Adrenergic stimulation results in a decrease in the cellular level of cAMP and enhanced release of mediators (Kaliner et al., 1972). Cholinergic stimulation of lung fragments with picomolar concentrations of carbachol results in a marked enhancement of SRS-A release and a moderate enhancement of histamine release (Kaliner et al., 1972). The demonstration that this effect can be blocked with atropine and the observation that the α-adrenergic and the cholinergic effects are additive indicate that these are unique mechanisms of enhancement (Kaliner et al., 1972). Cholinergic stimulation of other tissues has produced an increase in level of cyclic guanosine 3′,5′-monophosphate (cGMP) (Ferrendelli et al., 1970; Kuo et al., 1972), and these observations plus the ability of 8-bromo-cGMP to enhance the release of both histamine and SRS-A suggest that cholinergic stimulation of human lung fragments enhances the antigen-induced release of both mediators by increasing the tissue level of cGMP.

3.4. In Vivo Production

Indirect evidence indicates that the in vivo release of SRS-A is an important component of inflammatory reactions involving bronchial smooth muscle constriction and increased vascular permeability in certain species. Two experimental models of *in vivo* release of SRS-A have been described. The *in vivo* activity of this mediator in the rat model has not been defined. Continuing studies in the guinea pig indicate a unique mechanism of action for SRS-A (Drazen and Austen, 1974).

3.4.1. Rat Peritoneal Cavity

The observation by Rapp (1961) that SRS-A was released in the peritoneal cavity of rats prepared with a heterologous antibody–antigen system was the first evidence for *in vivo* production and release of this mediator. Since this initial observation, subsequent studies have demonstrated that rat antibody of the IgGa class (Stechschulte *et al.*, 1967; Morse *et al.*, 1968) and a second rat antibody, IgE antibody (Stechschulte *et al.*, 1970*b*; Orange *et al.*, 1970), are capable of preparing the rat peritoneal cavity for the release of both histamine and SRS-A. The failure to obtain SRS-A release in the face of significant amounts of histamine release in animals sacrificed prior to antigen challenge has not been explained. It is also of interest that IgGa and IgE antibodies have distinctly different optimum periods of sensitization for the passive cutaneous anaphylactic (PCA) reaction and for the release of histamine in the peritoneal cavity. However, both antibodies have a short latent period in the peritoneal cavity for preparation of SRS-A release (Stechschulte *et al.*, 1967; Orange *et al.*, 1969*b*, 1970). The requirement for the polymorphonuclear leukocyte (PMN) in the antigen-induced release of SRS-A in the rat peritoneal cavity prepared with the IgGa antibody is based on the observation that marked suppression of SRS-A release occurs when circulating PMNs are depleted using either nitrogen mustard or rabbit antiserum directed against this cell type (Orange *et al.*, 1968). The presence of increased numbers of eosinophils or macrophages suppresses the release of SRS-A (Orange and Austen, 1969*b*; Orange *et al.*, 1969*b*). The reaction pathway for release of SRS-A requuires the presence of an intact complement system (Orange *et al.*, 1968). In contrast, IgE antibody utilizes the mast cell for the release of both histamine and SRS-A (Orange *et al.*, 1969*b*, 1970) and does not require an intact complement system. Destruction of mast cells by i.p. administration of distilled water or antisera directed against this cell population results in complete inhibition of both histamine and SRS-A release. The rat peritoneal cavity has provided a means for the *in vivo* production of large quantities of SRS-A for purification and characterization studies of this molecule (Orange *et al.*, 1973). The cells and tissues obtained from this cavity have not successfully been adapted for the *in vitro* dissection of the reaction pathway leading to the release of this molecule.

3.4.2. Guinea Pig Circulation

The observation that the SRS-A adsorbed to serum proteins could be fully recovered by ethanol extraction (Orange and Austen, 1969*a*), plus the development of techniques for purification and characterization of this molecule (Orange et al., 1973), permitted the detection of SRS-A during systemic anaphylaxis in the guinea pig (Stechschulte et al., 1973). The presence of SRS-A in circulation after i.v. antigen challenge of sensitized guinea pigs was first noted at 1 min, with peak concentrations of 25–60 units of SRS-A/ml of plasma being detected at 4–7 min after antigen challenge. Pretreatment of these animals with mepyramine maleate prevented the characteristic sneezing, coughing, and scratching seen in guinea pig anaphylaxis but did not prevent their demise within 4–10 min. These observations add circulating SRS-A to the list of mediators known to be released during systemic anaphylaxis in the guinea pig. Since a histamine antagonist does not prevent death in these animals and the i.v. injection of SRS-A does not cause death in normal animals (Drazen and Austen, 1974), additional investigations will be required to define the effects of in vivo SRS-A release.

4. CONCLUDING COMMENTS

"Slow reacting substance of anaphylaxis" (SRS-A) and "slow reacting substance" (SRS) were originally descriptions of an in vitro stimulator activity on the guinea pig ileum detected in tissue perfusates after antigen and 48/80 challenge, respectively. This biological activity which is generated by different techniques has been extensively investigated in a number of laboratories and appears to have identical physicochemical properties. Although its chemical structure is unknown, the biological activity can be described as a highly potent, low molecular weight, acidic molecule which is distinct from the other recognized chemical mediators. This molecule has known in vivo effects on vascular permeability and respiratory dynamics, and the former effect makes it a potential contributor to any inflammatory reaction.

5. REFERENCES

Ambache, N., 1966, Biological characterization of, and structure–action studies on, smooth-muscle-contracting hydroxy-acids, Mem. Soc. Endocrinol. 14:19.

Amdur, M. O., and Mead, J., 1958, Mechanics of respiration in unanesthetized guinea pigs, Am. J. Physiol. 192:364.

Änggard, E., and Samuelsson, B., 1965, Biosynthesis of prostaglandins from arachidonic acid in guinea pig lung, J. Biol. Chem 240:3518.

Änggard, E., Bergqvist, U., Högberg, B., Johansson, K., Thon, I. L., and Uvnäs, B., 1963, Biologically active principles occurring on histamine release from cat paw, guinea pig lung and isolated rat mast cells, Acta Physiol. Scand. 59:97.

Assem, E. S. K., and Mongar, J. L., 1970, Inhibition of allergic reactions in man and other species by cromoglycate, *Int. Arch. Allergy Appl. Immunol.* **38:**68.

Austen, K. F., 1973, A review of immunological, biochemical, and pharmacological factors in the release of chemical mediators from human lung, in: *Asthma: Physiology, Immunopharmacology, and Treatment* (K. F. Austen and L. M. Lichtenstein, eds.), p. 71, Academic Press, New York.

Austen, K. F., and Brocklehurst, W. E., 1961, Anaphylaxis in chopped guinea pig lung. II. Enhancement of the anaphylactic release of histamine and slow reacting substance by certain dibasic aliphatic acids and inhibition by monobasic fatty acids, *J. Exp. Med.* **113:**541.

Becker, E. L., 1959, *In vitro* models for the allergic reaction, in: *Mechanisms of Hypersensitivity* (J. H. Shaffer, G. A. Logrippo, and M. W. Chase, eds.), p. 305, Little, Brown, Boston.

Berry, P. A., and Collier, H. O. J., 1964, Bronchoconstrictor action and antagonism of a slow reacting substance from anaphylaxis of guinea pig isolated lung, *Brit. J. Pharmacol. Chemother.* **23:**201.

Berry, P. A., Collier, H. O. J., and Holgate, J. A., 1963, Bronchoconstrictor action *in vivo* of slow reacting substance in anaphylaxis (SRS-A) and its antagonism, *J. Physiol. (Lond.)* **165:**41P.

Boreus, L. O., and Chakravarty, N., 1960, Tissue mast cells, histamine and "slow-reacting substance" in anaphylactic reaction in guinea pig, *Acta Physiol. Scand.* **48:**315.

Brocklehurst, W. E., 1953, Occurrence of an unidentified substance during anaphylactic shock in cavy lung, *J. Physiol. (Lond.)* **120:**16P.

Brocklehurst, W. E., 1960, The release of histamine and formation of a slow reacting substance (SRS-A) during anaphylactic shock, *J. Physiol. (Lond.)* **151:**416.

Brocklehurst, W. E., 1962, Slow reacting substance and related compounds, *Prog. Allergy* **6:**539.

Brocklehurst, W. E., 1963, "SRS-A": The slow reacting substance of anaphylaxis, *Biochem. Pharmacol.* **12:**431.

Brocklehurst, W. E., and Mawer, G. E., 1966, The purification of a kininogen from human plasma, *Brit. J. Pharmacol.* **27:**256.

Chakravarty, N., 1959*a*, A method for the assay of "slow reacting substance," *Acta Physiol. Scand.* **46:**298.

Chakravarty, N., 1959*b*, Observations on histamine release and formation of a lipid soluble smooth-muscle stimulating principle ("SRS") by antigen–antibody reaction and compound 48/80, academic thesis (Stockholm).

Chakravarty, N., 1960, The occurrence of a lipid-soluble smooth-muscle stimulating principle ("SRS") in anaphylaxis, *Acta Physiol. Scand.* **48:**167.

Chakravarty, N., and Uvnäs, B., 1959, Histamine and a lipid-soluble smooth-muscle stimulating principle ("SRS") in anaphylactic reaction, *Acta Physiol. Scand.* **48:**302.

Chakravarty, N., Högberg, B., and Uvnäs, B., 1959, Mechanism of release by compound 48/80 of histamine and of a lipid-soluble smooth muscle stimulating principle ("SRS"), *Acta Physiol. Scand.* **45:**255.

Chang, M. M., and Leeman, S. E., 1970, Isolation of a sialogogic peptide from bovine hypothalamic tissue and its characterization as substance P, *J. Biol. Chem.* **245:**4784.

Charlwood, P. A., and Gordon, A. H., 1958, Electrophoresis in a density gradient, *Biochem. J.* **70:**433.

Cirstea, M., Niculescu, V., Rusovici, L., and Suhaciu, G. L., 1967, Sialic acids and slow reacting substance of anaphylaxis (SRS-A), *Int. Arch. Allergy* **32:**105.

Clements, J. A., Jones, A. L., Felts, J. M., and Gould, K. G., Jr., 1972, Dispersal of rabbit lung into individual viable cells: A new model for the study of lung metabolism, *Science* 178:1209.

Curry, J. J., and Lowell, F. C., 1948, Measurement of vital capacity in asthmatic subjects receiving histamine and acetyl-beta-methyl choline, *J. Allergy* 19:9.

Dale, H. H., and Laidlaw, P. P., 1910, The physiological action of β-imidazolyl-ethylamine, *J. Physiol. (Lond.)* 41:318.

Drazen, J. M., and Austen, K. F., 1974, Effects of intravenous administration of slow-reacting substance of anaphylaxis, histamine, bradykinin and prostaglandin $F_{2\alpha}$ on pulmonary mechanics in the guinea pig, *J. Clin. Invest.* 53:1679.

Feldberg, W., and Kellaway, C. H., 1938, Liberation of histamine and formation of lysolecithin-like substance by cobra venom, *J. Physiol. (Lond.)* 94:187.

Ferrendelli, J. A., Steiner, A. L., McDougal, D. R., and Kipnis, D. M., 1970, The effect of oxotremorine and atropine on cGMP and cAMP levels in mouse cerebral cortex and cerebellum, *Biochem Biophys. Res. Commun.* 41:1061.

Grant, J. A., and Lichtenstein, L. M., 1974, Release of slow reacting substance of anaphylaxis from human leukocytes, *J. Immunol.* 112:897.

Herxheimer, H., and Stresemann, E., 1963, The effect of slow reacting substance (SRS-A) in guinea pigs and in asthmatic patients, *J. Physiol. (Lond.)* 165:78p.

Ishizaka, T., Ishizaka, K., Orange, R. P., and Austen, K. F., 1971, The capacity of human immunoglobulin E to mediate the release of histamine and slow reacting substance of anaphylaxis (SRS-A) from monkey lung, *J. Immunol.* 104:335.

Ishizaka, T., Ishizaka, K., and Tomioka, H., 1972, Release of histamine and slow reacting substance of anaphylaxis (SRS-A) by anti IgE reactions on monkey mast cells, *J. Immunol.* 108:513.

Kaliner, M., Orange, R. P., and Austen, K. F., 1972, Immunological release of histamine and slow reacting substance of anaphylaxis from human lung. IV. Enhancement by cholinergic and alpha adrenergic stimulation, *J. Exp. Med.* 136:556.

Kay, A. B., and Austen, K. F., 1971, The IgE-mediated release of a eosinophil leukocyte chemotactic factor from human lung, *J. Immunol.* 107:899.

Kuo, J., Lee, T., Reyes, P. L., Watton, K. G., Donnelly, T. E., Jr., and Greengard, P., 1972, Cyclic nucleotide–dependent protein kinases. X. An assay method for the measurement of guanosine 3′,5′ monophosphate in various biological materials and a study of agents regulating its levels in heart and brain, *J. Biol. Chem.* 247:16.

Kellaway, C. H., and Trethewie, E. R., 1940, The liberation of slow reacting smooth muscle-stimulating substance in anaphylaxis, *Quart. J. Exp. Physiol.* 30:121.

Konzett, H., and Rössler, R., 1940, Versuchsanordnung zer Untersuchugen an der Bronchiolmuskulatur, *Naunyn-Schmiedebergs Arch. Exp. Pathol. Pharmakol.* 195:71.

Lembeck, F., and Zetler, G., 1971, *IEPT, Pharmacology of Naturally Occurring Polypeptides and Lipid-Soluble Acids,* Vol. 1, p. 29, Pergamon, Oxford.

Lewis, R. A., Wasserman, S. I., Goetzl, E. J., and Austen, K. F., 1974, Immunological release of chemical mediators from isolated human lung cells, *Clin. Res.* 22:422A.

Mongar, J. L., and Schild, H. O., 1962, Cellular mechanisms in anaphylaxis, *Physiol. Rev.* 42:2.

Morse, H. C., III, Bloch, K. J., and Austen, K. F., 1968, Biologic properties of rat antibodies. II. Time-course of appearance of antibodies involved in antigen-induced release of slow reacting substance of anaphylaxis (SRS-A): Association of this activity with rat IgGa, *J. Immunol.* 101:658.

Orange, R. P., 1974, Dissociation of the *in vitro* immunologic release of histamine and slow reacting substance of anaphylaxis (SRS-A) from human lung using cytochalasins A and B, *Fed. Proc.* 33:761.

Orange, R. P., and Austen, K. F., 1969*a,* Slow reacting substance of anaphylaxis, *Advan. Immunol.* **10**:105.

Orange, R. P., and Austen, K. F., 1969*b,* Slow reacting substance of anaphylaxis in the rat, in: *Cellular and Humoral Mechanisms in Anaphylaxis and Allergy* (H. Z. Movat, ed.), p. 196, Karger, Basel and New York.

Orange, R. P., and Austen, K. F., 1971, The immunologic release of chemical mediators of immediate-type hypersensitivity from human lung, in: *Progress in Immunology,* p. 173, Academic Press, New York.

Orange, R. P., and Austen, K. F., 1974, The biological assay of slow reacting substances, in: *Methods in Immunology and Immunochemistry* (C. A. Williams, ed.), in press, Rockefeller University Press, New York.

Orange, R. P., Valentine, M. D., and Austen, K. F., 1968, Antigen-induced release of slow reacting substance of anaphylaxis (SRS-A) in rats prepared with homologous antibody, *J. Exp. Med.* **127**:767.

Orange, R. P., Ishizaka, T., Ishizaka, K., Karnovsky, M. L., and Austen, K. F., 1969*a,* Pharmacologic characterization of slow reacting substance of anaphylaxis (SRS-A), *Fed. Proc.* **28**:678.

Orange, R. P., Stechschulte, D. J., and Austen, K. F., 1969*b,* Cellular mechanisms involved in the release of slow reacting substance of anaphylaxis, *Fed. Proc.* **28**:1710.

Orange, R. P., Stechschulte, D. J., and Austen, K. F., 1970, Immunologic and biologic properties of rat IgE. II. Capacity to mediate the immunologic release of histamine and slow-reacting substance of anaphylaxis (SRS-A), *J. Immunol.* **105**:1087.

Orange, R. P., Austen, W. G., and Austen, K. F., 1971, Immunological release of histamine and slow reacting substance of anaphylaxis from human lung. I. Modulation by agents influencing cellular levels of cyclic 3',5'-adenosine monophosphate, *J. Exp. Med.* **134**:136s.

Orange, R. P., Murphy, R. C., Karnovsky, M. D., and Austen, K. F., 1973, The physicochemical characteristics and purification of slow reacting substance of anaphylaxis, *J. Immunol.* **110**:760.

Ovary, Z., Benacerraf, B., and Bloch, K. F., 1963, Properties of guinea pig 7S antibodies. II. Identification of antibodies involved in passive cutaneous and systemic anaphylaxis, *J. Exp. Med.* **117**:951.

Parish, W. E., 1967, Release of histamine and slow reacting substance with mast cell changes after challenge of human lung sensitized passively with reagin *in vitro, Nature (Lond.)* **215**:738.

Parish, W. E., 1973, A human heat-stable anaphylactic or anaphylactoid antibody which may participate in pulmonary disorders, in: *Asthma: Physiology, Immunopharmacology, and Treatment* (K. F. Austen and L. M. Lichtenstein, eds.), p. 71, Academic Press, New York.

Paton, W. D. M., 1951, Compound 48/80: A potent histamine liberator, *Brit. J. Pharmacol.* **6**:499.

Piper, P. J., and Vane, J. R., 1969, Release of additional factors in anaphylaxis and its antagonism by anti-inflammatory drugs, *Nature (Lond.)* **223**:29.

Rapp, H. J., 1961, The release of a slow reacting substance (SRS) in the peritoneal cavity of rats by antigen–antibody interaction, *J. Physiol. (Lond.)* **158**:35P.

Schild, H. O., 1936, Histamine release and anaphylactic shock in isolated lungs of guinea pigs, *Quart. J. Exp. Physiol.* **26**:165.

Sheard, P., and Blair, A. M. J. N., 1970, Disodium cromoglycate: Activity in three *in vitro* models of the immediate hypersensitivity reaction in lung, *Int. Arch. Allergy Appl. Immunol.* **38**:217.

Sheard, P., Killingback, P. G., and Blair, A. M. J. N., 1967, Antigen induced release of histamine and SRS-A from human lung passively sensitized with reaginic serum, *Nature (Lond.)* 216:283.

Stechschulte, D. J., Austen, K. F., and Bloch, K. J., 1967, Antibodies involved in the antigen-induced release of slow reacting substance of anaphylaxis (SRS-A) in the guinea pig and rat, *J. Exp. Med.* 125:127.

Stechschulte, D. J., Orange, R. P., and Austen, K. F., 1970a, Two immunochemically distinct homologous antibodies capable of mediating immediate hypersensitivity reactions in the rat, mouse and guinea pig, in: *New Concepts in Allergy and Clinical Immunology*, p. 245, Excerpta Medica International Congress Series No. 232, Excerpta Medica, Amsterdam

Stechschulte, D. J., Orange, R. P., and Austen, K. F., 1970b, Immunologic and biologic properties of rat IgE. I. Immunochemical identification of rat IgE, *J. Immunol.* 105:1082.

Stechschulte, D. J., Orange, R. P., and Austen, K. F., 1973, Detection of slow reacting substance of anaphylaxis (SRS-A) in plasma of guinea pigs during anaphylaxis, *J. Immunol.* 111:1585.

Strandberg, K., 1971a, Release of histamine and formation of slow reacting substance in the cat paw induced by compound 48/80, *Acta Physiol. Scand.* 82:47.

Strandberg, K., 1971b, Histamine and SRS in cat paw, *Acta Physiol. Scand.* 82:509.

Strandberg, K., and Uvnäs, B., 1971, Purification and properties of SRS, *Acta Physiol. Scand.* 82:358.

Vogt, W., 1957, Pharmacologically active substances formed in egg yolk by cobra venom, *J. Physiol. (Lond.)* 136:131.

Vogt, W., 1958, Naturally occurring lipid-soluble acids of pharmacological interest, *Pharmacol. Rev.* 10:407.

Vogt, W., 1969, Slow reacting substances, in: *Cellular and Humoral Mechanisms of Anaphylaxis and Allergy* (H. Z. Movat, ed.), p. 197, Karger, New York.

Vogt, W., Meyer, U., Kunze, H., Lufft, E., and Babille, S., 1969, Entstehung von SRS-C in der durchströmten Meerschweinchenlunge durch Phospholipase A, *Naunyn-Schmiedebergs Arch. Exp. Path. Pharmakol.* 262:124.

von Euler, U. S., and Gaddum, J. H., 1931, An unidentified depressor substance in certain tissue extracts, *J. Physiol. (Lond.)* 72:74.

INDEX